Synopsis of Cardiac Physical Diagnosis

Synopsis of Cardiac Physical Diagnosis

Second Edition

Jonathan Abrams, M.D.

Professor of Medicine, Division of Cardiology, The University of New Mexico School of Medicine, Albuquerque

Foreword by

John Michael Criley, M.D., M.A.C.P., F.A.C.C.
Professor Emeritus of Medicine and Radiological Sciences, University of California, Los Angeles, School of Medicine

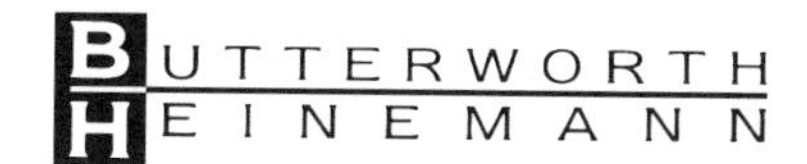

Boston Oxford Auckland Johannesburg Melbourne New Delhi

Every effort has been made to ensure that the drug dosage schedules within this text are accurate and conform to standards accepted at time of publication. However, as treatment recommendations vary in the light of continuing research and clinical experience, the reader is advised to verify drug dosage schedules herein with information found on product information sheets. This is especially true in cases of new or infrequently used drugs.

 Recognizing the importance of preserving what has been written, Butterworth–Heinemann prints its books on acid-free paper whenever possible.

Library of Congress Cataloging-in-Publication Data

Abrams, Jonathan.
Synopsis of cardiac physical diagnosis / Jonathan Abrams.—2nd ed.
p. ; cm.
Includes bibliographical references and index.
ISBN 0-7506-7338-9 (alk. paper)
1. Heart—Sounds. 2. Heart—Diseases—Diagnosis. 3. Physical diagnosis. I. Title.
[DNLM: 1. Heart Diseases—diagnosis. 2. Heart Function Tests. WG 141 A161e 2001]
RC683.5.A9 A27 2001
616.1'20754—dc21 00-066797

British Library Cataloguing-in-Publication Data
A catalogue record for this book is available from the British Library.

The publisher offers special discounts on bulk orders of this book.
For information, please contact:

Manager of Special Sales
Butterworth–Heinemann
225 Wildwood Avenue
Woburn, MA 01801-2041
Tel: 781-904-2500
Fax: 781-904-2620

For information on all Butterworth–Heinemann publications available, contact our World Wide Web home page at: http://www.bh.com

10 9 8 7 6 5 4 3 2

Printed in the United States of America

Contents

Foreword

Jonathan Abrams was greatly influenced by master clinicians from the golden era of clinical cardiology, and, as a result, is a superb diagnostician who is fully conversant with the old as well as the new technology. He has placed the value of the old and the new in proper perspective in this eminently readable tome. The golden era reached its apogee in the mid-20th century through the observations, writings, and teachings of W. Proctor Harvey, Paul Wood, Aubrey Leatham, Noble Fowler, Ernest Craige, Abe Ravin, and others who inspired and nurtured Dr. Abrams' long interest in the bedside cardiovascular examination.

Cardiac physical examination is an ancient technology and is and was a blend of art and science. In its infancy, it was principally art supported by scant science. William Harvey's discovery of the true nature of circulation was a most important first step in establishing a scientific foothold, and Laennec's seminal observations following his 1819 invention of the stethoscope greatly increased the precision of the bedside evaluation of the cardiac patient. Clinical-pathologic correlations by clinicians in the 19th century and first half of the 20th century greatly added to our understanding of causation of physical findings and led to a plethora of eponyms: Corrigan's and Quincke's pulses, Austin Flint's and Graham Steell's murmurs, and Osler's nodes and Fallot's tetralogy are permanent fixtures in our nosology. According to Peter Mere Latham in 1847, "we were never tired of visiting and examining and ausculting, and of examining and ausculting again and again."

The last half of the 20th century yielded a virtual cornucopia of modalities that, by all rights, should have advanced interest in the cardiac examination to a degree that could not have been imagined by prior generations of clinicians. Instead of waiting for the patient's demise and the performance of necropsy, contemporary clinicians are able to hone their skills by correlating their bedside findings with cardiac echo-Doppler ultrasonography, electron beam or magnetic resonance tomography, or cardiac catheterization and angiography. This dazzling array of technology provided a scientific basis for the understanding of cardiac physical findings. Unfortunately this infusion of science has not enhanced interest in the cardiac physical examination, but sadly has served to supplant and ultimately degrade it.

The academic literature is replete with reports of poor performance in cardiac auscultation among medical trainees and their recently trained instructors, a formula for perpetuation of mediocrity in the future. When "the Blues Brothers" (a.k.a. Blue Cross and Blue Shield) and other third-party payers discontinued reimbursement for phonocardiography, the handwriting on the wall clearly articulated that the diagnostic value of understanding and documenting heart sounds and murmurs had been upstaged and supplanted by high technology. Unfortunately, these studies are often interpreted by persons unaware of the patient's symptoms, signs, and clinical examination. Requisitions for echocardiography may merely read "evaluate murmur," and the interpreter is often happy to oblige with an interpretation that justifies the study.

Jonathan Abrams puts the old and the new into proper perspective in this compendium of bedside cardiac physical findings, supported by newly gained knowledge of the underlying mechanisms. The text is replete with practical and useful information that should restore interest, and enhance the skill level, in the bedside evaluation of the patient with cardiovascular physical findings. The art and science of bedside cardiac evaluation have a glorious past and deserve the respect afforded by Dr. Abrams.

John Michael Criley

Preface

In this age of technology it is increasingly difficult to emphasize and teach physical diagnosis as a skill for physicians and health care professionals. Doppler-echocardiography has become a routine diagnostic tool in the evaluation of individuals with possible, suspect, or known cardiovascular disease. Too often the echo results circumvent the perceived need of the examiner to perform a careful and complete cardiac physical examination. All that is necessary appears to be revealed by the ubiquitous echo report.

This monograph, then, flies in the face of present reality by providing a detailed guide to the normal and abnormal cardiac physical examination in adults. Review and synthesis of this material should enable the examiner to conduct a thorough and accurate assessment of the cardiovascular system in health and disease.

The genesis of this book is my original text, *Essentials of Cardiac Physical Diagnosis*, published by Lea and Febiger in 1987, and the shorter *Synopsis of Cardiac Physical Diagnosis*, published in 1989. Both volumes have been too long out of print. The present book is essentially a second edition of the original *Synopsis*, moderately pared down, but fundamentally similar.

I would like to express my deep appreciation to Susan Pioli of Butterworth-Heinemann, who graciously approved this new edition. Joseph Alpert, the chair of medicine at the University of Arizona School of Medicine, and an outstanding clinical cardiologist, is in part responsible for this publication through his support and guidance in helping me find a new publisher. Thanks Joe!

Jonathan Abrams

Part I

Basic Principles of Cardiovascular Physical Diagnosis: The Approach to the Patient

1

Cardiac Auscultation: Cardiac Sound, Cardiac Cycle, and the Stethoscope

Pertinent Features of Cardiac Sound

Several important features of cardiac sound require analysis during auscultation. *Loudness* of sound is a subjective judgment, closely related to the amplitude or intensity of sound waves. The *pitch* of a heart sound or murmur relates to the underlying *frequency.* Soft, rough, low-frequency sounds are low pitched (25–150 Hz), whereas high-frequency sounds are high pitched. The *quality* or tone of a sound relates to the combination of waveform contours, harmonics, and overtones.

For most persons, the audible range of cardiac sound is approximately 30–80 Hz, although the human ear is capable of detecting sound vibrations as high as 16,000–18,000 Hz. The optimal range of auditory acuity is 1000–2000 Hz, which is higher than the range of most cardiac sound. Most cardiac sound is low frequency (less than 150 Hz). Very low-frequency events (less than 25 Hz) are inaudible but often may be palpable; this explains the occasional finding of palpable atrial and ventricular filling sounds (S_4 and S_3) in individuals in whom these components are inaudible.

In general, anything between the stethoscope and the heart such as adipose tissue, breast, muscular tissue, or lung parenchyma with increased air will attenuate cardiac sound. Lean individuals with little excess body tissue tend to have louder heart sounds and murmurs.

Background Noise

Often unnoticed environmental noise can prevent the detection of heart murmurs, particularly those of high frequency. The level of noise in hospital rooms, clinics, or the typical examining room is 60–75 dB, well above the optimal (but impractical) level of 35 dB. If there is an unusual amount of noise (auto or air traffic, construction, human conversation) in the examining area, higher frequency sounds and murmurs may be inaudible even to the most experienced clinicians.

Presbycusis

Young people normally hear high-frequency sounds better than older people. With aging, a selective high-frequency hearing loss is common. Fortunately, this has no important impact on auscultation because most cardiac sound is in the low–medium-frequency range.

Theory of Heart Sound Production

It is generally accepted that cardiac sounds represent vibrations of cardiac structures and blood within the heart. These vibrations are produced by the acceleration or deceleration of the blood mass during the cardiac cycle. In the past, cardiac sounds were thought to originate from the valves themselves; however, normal valve tissue is not rigid or thick enough to produce sound solely due to leaflet apposition. Rather, the tensing of the closed valves resulting from rapidly increasing pressure gradients produces sound vibrations. The pressure "crossover" initiating S_1 or S_2 (e.g., left atrial–left ventricular, aorta–left ventricular) always precedes the heart sound itself (Figure 1-1). Blood flow continues in the face of a pressure "gradient" as a result of inertial forces. Therefore, the valve leaflets still are in motion at the precise point of pressure crossover (see Figure 6-1).

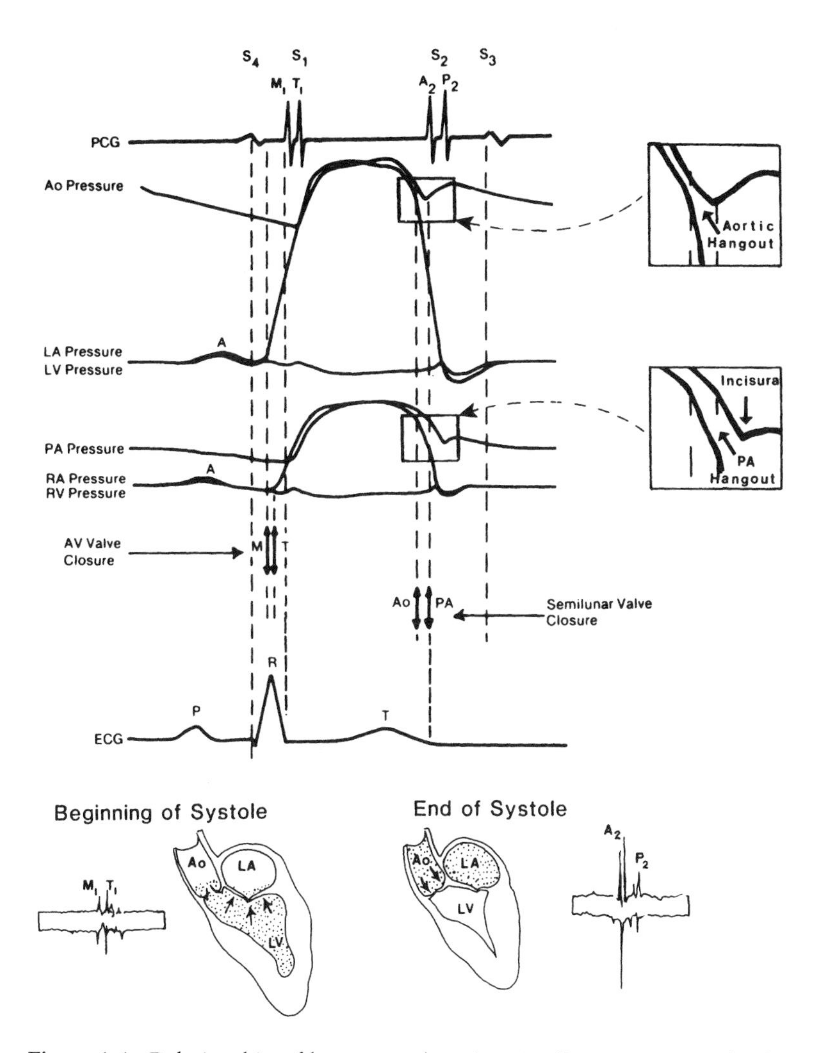

Figure 1-1. Relationship of heart sounds to intracardiac pressures and valve motion. See text for further discussion.

Cardiac sound, whether normal or abnormal, results from abrupt accelerating or decelerating forces that stretch the surrounding cardiac structures to their elastic limits. The more rapid these forces, the louder is the sound and the higher is the frequency. Low-frequency sound (S_3, S_4) typically reflects large amounts of blood moving at low velocity.

The Cardiac Cycle

The four heart sounds are intimately related to electromechanical events within the heart. To make any sense of auscultation, one must understand the basic sequence of the cardiac cycle, which is comprised of *systole,* the ventricular ejection phase, and *diastole,* the ventricular relaxation and filling phase.

Systole

Electrical activation of the ventricles is initiated by the QRS of the electrocardiogram. Depolarization of the left ventricle (LV) begins before that in the right ventricle (RV). The rapidly rising pressure in each ventricle helps close the two AV valves, resulting in the first heart sound, S_1 (see Chapter 5). However, because the LV has a far greater muscle mass and must develop a peak systolic pressure four to five times greater than the RV, it takes longer for isovolumic pressure in the LV to open the aortic valve than for RV pressure to open the pulmonary valve (isovolumic contraction time). Therefore, although LV electrical activation begins before the RV, pulmonary valve opening and ejection of blood into the pulmonary artery begin before aortic valve opening and ejection into the aorta (see Figure 1-1).

Diastole

During inspiration, aortic valve closure (A_2) occurs before pulmonary valve closure (P_2), but during expiration the two valves normally close simultaneously (see Figure 1-1 and Chapter 5). Pressure continues to fall in both ventricles after semilunar valve closure (isovolumic relaxation); the AV valves open passively (and silently) in early diastole when ventricular pressure drops below that in the corresponding atrium. The mitral valve opens before the tricuspid valve.

Rapid ventricular filling follows the maximal opening excursion of the mitral and tricuspid valves in diastole and results in the third heart sound, S_3 (see Chapter 6). Approximately 70–80% of the ventricular end-diastolic volume is achieved during early and middiastole, well before atrial contraction. The AV valves drift back toward their respective atria with a closing motion in mid diastole. Following the P wave, the atria contract and the AV valves reopen, resulting in augmentation of blood flow into the ventricles in late diastole (S_4). At end diastole, the AV valves again begin a closing movement (see Figure 6-1). The mitral and tricuspid valves close completely with the onset of ventricular contraction. Ventricular-atrial pressure crossover, however, precedes actual AV valve closure by 25–50 msec (see Figure 1-1).

The Stethoscope

Knowledge of cardiac sound characteristics and their relationship to stethoscope design should be helpful to physicians motivated to obtain the maximum information from auscultation. Although the choice of stethoscope design and manufacturer is relatively limited, it is useful to examine the acoustic and practical characteristics of this indispensable instrument, such as sound transmission, frequency filtration, masking, and interference.

The stethoscope consists of a dual *chest piece* with a valve that allows switching from bell to diaphragm, *binaural connectors,* and *earpieces.* The component parts should be well made, durable, with no air leaks, and easy to use. A good stethoscope does not distort cardiac sound.

The Bell

The bell (Figure 1-2) is used primarily for detection of low-frequency sound (30–150 Hz). *Lower frequencies are attenuated, and higher-frequency sound is accentuated as increased pressure is applied to the bell.* Firm pressure with the bell stretches the skin of the chest wall, which transmits higher frequency sound vibrations; the bell then performs similarly to the diaphragm of the stethoscope. *Practical Point. To emphasize detection of low-frequency sounds (e.g., S_3, S_4, mitral rumble), the lightest possible contact pressure should be used with the bell.*

The bell should have a large diameter (at least 1 inch), a trumpet-shaped internal construction, and be relatively shallow. A detachable rubber ring is highly desirable for use in conjunction with the bell (see

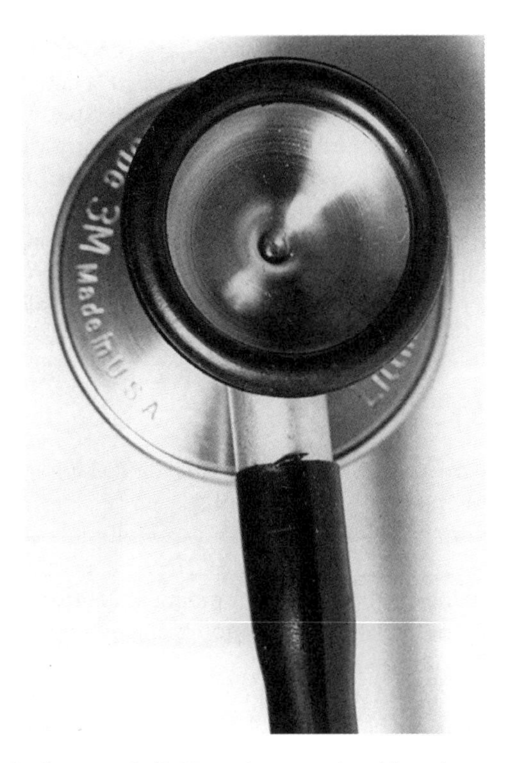

Figure 1-2. Stethoscope bell. Note the smooth rubber rim attached to the metallic bell. It is advisable to use a rubber ring with the stethoscope bell to provide a skin seal with light stethoscope pressure, thus increasing the ability to hear low-frequency cardiac sound.

Figure 1-2). This allows for light skin contact pressure, minimizes production of an air leak, increases the diameter of the bell, and does not get cold.

The Diaphragm

The diaphragm is the high-frequency component of the chest piece. A proper diaphragm should filter out low frequencies (less than 300 Hz); often, it will appear to amplify high-pitched cardiac sound. As with the bell, increasing pressure tightens the skin and allows transmission of higher frequency sound.

Earpieces and Binaurals

Probably the most common problem in stethoscope usage is improper fit of the binaurals and earpieces. Poor fit can result in decreased acuity in auscultation. Comfort is of primary importance. Large rather than small earpieces are best. Small earpieces can penetrate too far into the external ear canal and, by impinging against the ear canal wall, may even become occluded. *Practical Point: The use of a poorly fitting stethoscope will result in decreased acuity in cardiac auscultation.*

How to Use the Stethoscope

Identification of Systole and Diastole

Proper identification of the two phases of the cardiac cycle usually is not difficult. During tachycardia, however, diastole shortens more than systole; and with rapid heart rates, it may be difficult to distinguish between the two. When there are extra sounds (particularly an opening snap or midsystolic click), systole easily can be confused with diastole. If there are associated cardiac murmurs, the problem can be even more difficult. *Practical Point: Use the carotid pulse and apex impulse to identify the phases of the cardiac cycle. The carotid upstroke and the beginning outward thrust of the initial apex beat immediately follow S_1. S_2 occurs shortly after the carotid and apex impulses are felt* (Figure 1-3). S_2 normally is the louder of the two heart sounds heard at the base of the heart, an area that includes the second right and left interspace adjacent to the sternum.

"Inching"

Levine and Harvey popularized this valuable technique in which the stethoscope slowly is moved or inched from a site on the chest where systole and diastole are identified clearly to other precordial locations where it is more difficult to determine which sound is systolic or diastolic. By focusing on the characteristics of S_1 and S_2, the cadence of the cardiac cycle enables the observer to identify correctly systole and diastole at other precordial locations. It is best to begin auscultation at the base, where systole and diastole usually are most easily identified.

Selective Listening

Selective listening is the hallmark of accurate and meaningful cardiac auscultation. The importance of focusing on only one part of the

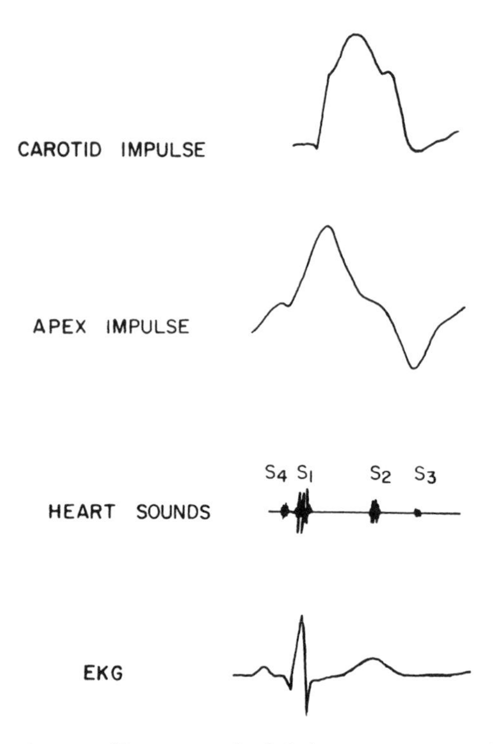

Figure 1-3. Timing of heart sounds. It is important to use simultaneous palpation of the carotid arterial pulse or the apical impulse when listening to the heart sounds. Note that S_1 immediately *precedes* the upstroke of the carotid pulse and is virtually simultaneous with the earliest palpable precordial activity. S_2 marks the end of systole and *follows* the palpable carotid and apical impulse.

cardiac cycle at a time during auscultation has been stressed by Dr. W. Proctor Harvey. For instance, when early systole is analyzed, only the acoustic events around S_1 are auscultated. The rest of systole and all of diastole are consciously excluded. Systole and diastole each should be divided into thirds—early, mid, and late—and each segment focused on in turn. Heart sounds should be assessed first, followed by attention to heart murmurs. With this approach, little will be missed. *Practical Point: Intense concentration is the key to competent cardiac auscultation.*

2

The Arterial Pulse

Examination of the arterial pulse often reveals valuable information about the cardiovascular system. In certain conditions, such as aortic valve disease, hypertrophic cardiomyopathy, and pericardial tamponade, an accurate assessment of pulse contour and amplitude can be of great importance in making a proper diagnosis. This chapter emphasizes how to extract the most data from careful *bedside examination* of the arterial pulse.

Normal Physiology

The arterial pulse wave is related to many physiologic factors, including the left ventricular stroke volume and ejection velocity as well as the relative compliance and capacity of the arterial system. The relative distensibility, or "stiffness," of the arterial system affects both the contour and velocity of the arterial pulse.

The first portion of the central aortic pulse wave (Figure 2-1) reflects the peak velocity of blood ejected during early systole, which is "stored" in the central aorta. The mid- to late-systolic portion of the normal pulse wave is produced by blood moving from the central aorta *to* the periphery simultaneously with a reflection of the pulse wave returning *from* the arteries of the upper body. With aging or decreased compliance of the arterial tree, the later portion of the pulse wave is accentuated, and the pulse contour becomes somewhat more sustained. A notch or change in slope on the early-pulse contour is called the *anacrotic notch* or *shoulder*.

Diastole is initiated by an abrupt negative wave called the *dicrotic notch* (see Figure 2-1). The nadir coincides precisely with aortic leaflet closure and the aortic component of S_2 (A_2). *Practical Point: The anacrotic and dicrotic notches normally cannot be felt. Do not expect to palpate them when examining the arterial pulse.* Normally, the arterial pulse is not palpable during diastole.

Pulse Wave Alteration in the Periphery

The normal pulse contour is altered with increasing distance from the aortic valve, characterized by a greater amplitude and velocity and a lower dicrotic notch; these changes become progressively more pronounced distally (Figure 2-2). *Practical Point: The peripheral arteries (e.g., radial, femoral) should not be used routinely to assess the arterial pulse contour. Normal physiologic pulse wave alteration in distal vessels may mask important diagnostic information present in the proximal vessels.* On the other hand, the augmented rate of rise and amplitude of the pulse in peripheral vessels increases the ability to

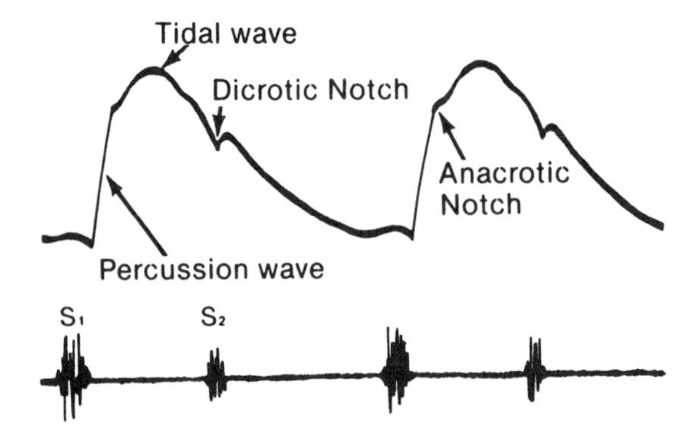

Figure 2-1. Normal arterial pulse. Note the rapid upstroke, the rounded summit or peak, and the falloff in late systole. Normally, only the systolic peak is palpable; diastolic events are not felt. The dicrotic notch times precisely with S_2 and coincident with aortic and pulmonic valve closure. The terms *percussion wave, tidal wave,* and *anacrotic notch* are discussed in the text.

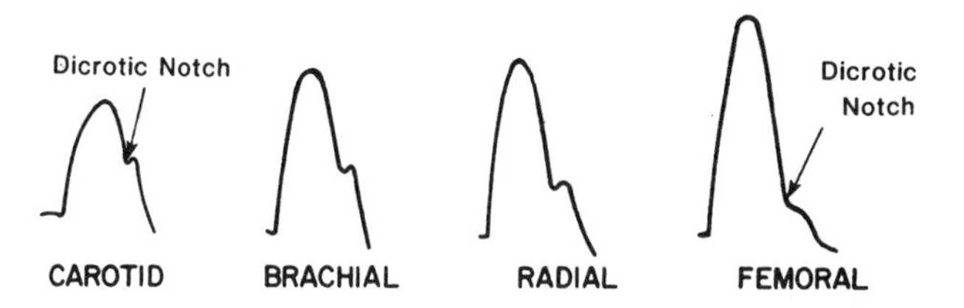

Figure 2-2. Arterial pulse contour alteration in the peripheral circulation. As the distance increases from the peripheral artery to the central aorta, the amplitude and upstroke velocity of the pulse contour also increase and the dicrotic notch becomes lower. The higher systolic pressure in peripheral arteries is one reason why the arterial pulse is best evaluated at the carotid artery rather than distally.

detect the subtle abnormalities of pulsus paradoxus and pulsus alternans (see later).

Pulse Wave Alterations with Decreased Vascular Compliance

In states of increased vascular resistance or stiffness, such as occurs with hypertension, the relatively noncompliant arterial tree contributes to increased pulse wave velocity. This increase results in a pulse contour with a rapid upstroke and greater amplitude. The thickened arterial walls of the aged or atherosclerotic subject may produce the same effect. Under such circumstances, a small or relatively normal LV stroke volume may be transmitted to the carotid with a brisk upstroke, giving a false-positive impression of the actual stroke volume. *Practical Point: In older subjects, hypertensive patients, or those with diffuse vascular disease, information obtained from examination of the arterial pulse is less reliable. By way of contrast, in the presence of intense arterial vasoconstriction, the palpable pulse volume may appear to be reduced when in fact the ejected stroke volume is normal.*

The Examination

Technique

Both the patient and the physician should be relaxed. The subject's head and thorax should be elevated slightly, at 15–30°. Either the thumb or the first two fingers are used to feel the arterial pulse; the finger pads usually are quite sensitive for optimal palpation. Gentle but firm pressure is necessary, with the thumb or finger placed directly on the summit of the vessel. To obtain maximal information, the palpating pressure should be varied. Surprisingly light pressure may be needed once direct contact with the blood vessel has been established. The normal pulse has a brief crest that is slightly sustained and somewhat rounded (see Figure 2-1).

Which Artery to Palpate?

In a complete cardiovascular examination, all accessible arterial pulses should be assessed. It is important to compare bilateral vessels. A missing or extremely weak pulse may have major significance, suggesting atherosclerosis, embolic occlusion, dissection, vascular compression, or a congenital anomaly. The brachial artery often is buried beneath the biceps muscle and may be difficult to localize. The right carotid artery may appear dilated in older subjects, particularly if there is hypertension; this usually is due to an innocuous kinking or buckling of the innominate vessels. In any patient with hypertension or in infants with heart failure, the radial or brachial artery and the femoral artery *must be palpated simultaneously* to exclude coarctation of the aorta. Normally, the femoral pulsation immediately precedes the radial pulse; in coarctation, the femoral arterial pulse is distinctly delayed and reduced in volume when compared to the arm pulses.

Use the Carotid Artery

The carotid arterial pulse provides the most accurate evaluation of the arterial pulse volume and contour because it is the largest palpable proximal vessel, the closest accessible artery to the aortic valve, and its contour closely resembles the directly recorded central aortic pulse. On the other hand, distal vessels may be affected by typical waveform alterations that occur in peripheral arteries (see Figure 2-2). Therefore, diagnostic abnormalities of the central arterial pulse may be attenuated or disappear in the peripheral circulation.

In examining the carotid artery, careful attention should be paid to the lower half of the neck. The adjacent sternocleidomastoid muscle should be under no tension, and pressure should not be placed on the carotid sinus itself.

Characteristics of the carotid arterial pulse include:

- Cardiac rhythm
- Pulse volume (generally related to the size of the stroke volume in the absence of vasoconstriction)
- Pulse amplitude
- Pulse contour, with special attention to the crest or peak of the pulse
- Speed or rate of rise of ejection (early systole)
- Stiffness or distensibility of the vessel wall

Occasionally one can feel a shudder or thrill in the carotid pulse representing a palpable bruit or transmitted murmur. Localized atherosclerosis or abnormalities of the left ventricular outflow tract account for most carotid thrills. A hyperkinetic circulation, often found in normal children or patients with aortic regurgitation, may produce a slight "buzz" to the carotid pulse. A loud murmur of ventricular septal defect or pulmonic stenosis occasionally radiates to the neck and produces a carotid thrill.

In older subjects or those in whom there is a suspicion of peripheral vascular disease, both the carotid and femoral arteries should be routinely auscultated and palpated. Some cardiac murmurs that intensify in the upper chest or clavicular areas and are well heard along the sternal edge are easily heard over the carotid arteries.

Abnormal Variants

Hyperkinetic Pulse

A hyperkinetic arterial pulse has a larger than normal amplitude and results from an increase in left ventricular ejection velocity, stroke volume, or arterial pressure. The pulse wave amplitude also may be augmented in persons with decreased arterial compliance, such as arterial wall thickening or systemic vasoconstriction. A hyperkinetic arterial pulse may result from cigarette smoking or any state of enhanced sympathetic activity; it is common in elderly subjects and usually implies an elevation in systolic blood pressure. Bounding or hyperkinetic pulses are typical of high output states, such as may be present with anxiety, anemia, thyrotoxicosis, exercise, a hot and humid environment, and alcohol intake.

Hypertension may cause a more forceful arterial pulse if the pulse wave velocity is increased, particularly if there is associated generalized arteriosclerosis. A hyperkinetic pulse is typical of aortic regurgitation where the runoff of the pulse may be very rapid, producing a bounding or collapsing pulse. Other high output states with increased distal arterial runoff, such as a patent ductus arteriosus, large AV fistulae, Paget's disease, or severe cirrhosis, may simulate the classic pulse of aortic regurgitation. In hypertrophic cardiomyopathy an early brisk pulse wave may be felt in the carotid arteries. In severe mitral regurgitation, the arterial pulse also may be brisk and tapping.

Hypokinetic Pulse

Small or diminished pulses are common in states of low cardiac output. A decreased left ventricular stroke volume results in a shorter left ventricular ejection time because there is less blood to eject. Impairment of LV function or overt congestive heart failure also is associated with a decreased velocity of ejection. Hypotensive states and LV outflow tract obstruction usually result in a small pulse volume. Intense vasoconstriction may reduce the pulse amplitude in the face of a normal stroke volume. *Practical Point: It is important to assess the rate of rise of the hypokinetic pulse. A normal upstroke (unsustained) indicates a decreased stroke volume without LV outflow obstruction, whereas a slow rising (sustained) pulse of small volume strongly suggests aortic stenosis.*

Pulsus Paradoxus

Pulsus paradoxus refers to a marked and exaggerated inspiratory fall in systolic blood pressure in which the palpable peripheral arterial pulse (and audible Korotkoff sounds) *disappear during inspiration.* This may give the impression of a cardiac arrhythmia, but the heartbeat is regular throughout. Paradoxus is a classic finding in pericardial tamponade (see later).

Because systolic arterial pressure normally falls slightly during inspiration, the word *paradoxus* actually is a misnomer, but its continued use is dictated by widespread use of this term. Normally, LV stroke volume decreases somewhat during inspiration because of diminished left heart filling; the inspiratory decrease in intrathoracic pressure causes pooling of blood in the pulmonary bed. Systemic arterial pressure therefore falls a few millimeters of mercury during inspiration. Right ventricular stroke volume, however, increases with inspiration. During expiration, this increased RV stroke volume is transmitted to the left heart, increasing LV stroke volume and systolic arterial pressure. The combination of these complex physiologic events results in modest respiration-related alterations in systolic blood pressure in normal subjects, which typically is undetectable on examination.

Inspiration normally reduces systolic arterial pressure less than 6–8 mmHg; if the inspiratory fall is more than 8 mmHg, pulsus paradoxus is said to be present. In general, however, the fall in inspiratory pressure should approach 10–12 mmHg before a definite diagnosis of abnormal physiology is made. In severe cases, the fall in blood pressure during inspiration may be 30–40 mmHg or more.

Causes

Several mechanisms result in abnormally large phasic alterations in RV and LV stroke volume during the respiratory cycle, which can produce a paradoxic pulse. *All such situations show a marked inspiratory decrease in LV filling.* The following conditions may be associated with pulsus paradoxus:

- Pericardial tamponade
- Asthma
- Emphysema
- Marked obesity
- Severe congestive heart failure
- Constrictive pericarditis

When paradox is detected, pericardial tamponade must be ruled out before other diagnoses are pursued.

Pericardial Tamponade

Pericardial tamponade is the most common and important cause of pulsus paradoxus. Detection of a paradoxic pulse may be the first or only clue to the underlying condition; recognition may be lifesaving. In pericardial tamponade, there is a marked inspiratory restricition of left ventricular filling and a fall in inspiratory LV stroke volume. Right ventricular stroke volume increases during inspiration; the additional RV blood reaches the LV during the next expiration and helps elevate systemic pressure. The RV actually may become compressed by the elevated pericardial pressure. Therefore, systolic arterial pressure and both RV and LV stroke volume fluctuate greatly during the respiratory cycle in pericardial tamponade. Large, noncompressive pericardial effusions usually do not produce a paradoxic pulse.

Asthma and Emphysema
A paradoxic pulse can be found in patients with severe obstructive lung disease as a result of exaggerated respiratory motion and wide swings in intrathoracic pressure. In such situations, pulsus paradoxus typically is modest (less than 15 mmHg) and unlikely to be palpable.

Marked Obesity
Paradoxic pulse has been reported in very obese patients, probably as a result of the increased work of breathing and large fluctuations in intrathoracic pressure.

Severe Congestive Heart Failure
A paradoxic pulse occasionally can be noted in some patients in heart failure. The enlarged heart is pulled inferiorly during inspiration, raising intrapericardial pressure and diminishing venous return.

Constrictive Pericarditis
A paradoxic pulse is found only occasionally in patients with pericardial constriction. It is a common misunderstanding that pulsus paradoxus is the rule in this condition. The obliterated pericardial space in constrictive pericarditis actually helps prevent marked respiratory alterations in ventricular filling from occurring.

Detection

Palpation Method
Light pressure with the fingers or thumb should be applied to a peripheral artery (e.g., brachial or radial) with careful attention to alterations of the pulse amplitude as related to the phases of the respiratory cycle.

Sphygmomanometer Method

To measure the actual magnitude of the paradoxic pulse, the blood pressure cuff should be inflated beyond peak systolic arterial pressure and then decompressed slowly and evenly at increments of no more than 4–5 mmHg at a time. Note (1) the pressure at which the first Korotkoff sounds appear during expiration, (2) the level when all beats become audible, and (3) the moment when the inspiratory and expiratory Korotkoff sounds become equally loud.

The degree of inspiratory decline is the difference between *initial* systolic arterial pressure (when the first Korotkoff sounds are heard during expiration) and the point at which *all* beats are well heard during *both* phases of respiration. Since a 4–6 mmHg fall in systemic arterial pressure is normal during inspiration, in subjects with a definite paradoxic pulse, the Korotkoff sounds will be inaudible or barely detectable during inspiration at a level more than 6–8 mmHg below peak systolic pressure and the pulse will seem grossly irregular. *To assess the presence of pulsus paradoxus, it is important to be sure the patient is breathing quietly and not hyperventilating or performing an inadvertent Valsalva maneuver.*

Arterial Pulse in Specific Cardiac Disorders

Examination of the arterial pulse can be helpful in establishing a diagnosis and assessing the severity of the underlying condition in a number of cardiovascular disorders.

Aortic Stenosis

In aortic stenosis (see Chapter 10), obstruction to LV ejection produces characteristic alterations of aortic pressure best detected in the carotid artery pulses (see Figure 2-3 and Table 10-1).

The carotid pulse in valvular aortic stenosis is *slow rising* (pulsus parvus), has a delayed peak (pulsus tardus or plateau pulse), is of small volume, exhibits a palpable thrill, and displays a prominent anacrotic notch. The decreased rate of rise is manifested by a "slow" or delayed upstroke. A sustained summit reflects the delayed peak. The small pulse volume is due to hemodynamic obstruction at valve level. A palpable thrill or shudder occurs near or on the arterial pulse

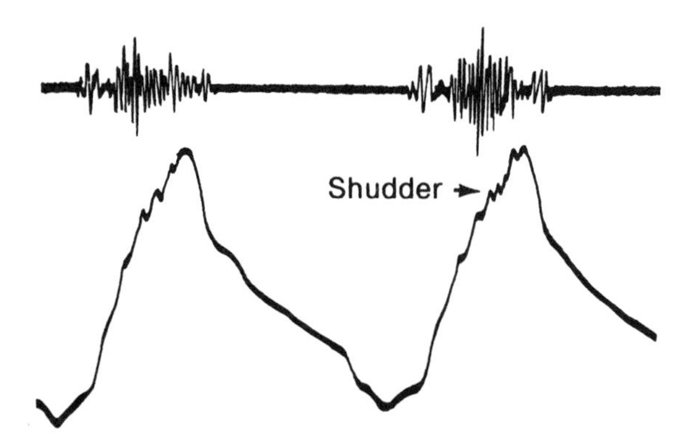

Figure 2-3. Arterial pulse in aortic stenosis. Note the delayed upstroke and the jagged contour representing a palpable shudder or transmitted thrill. The pulse volume usually is decreased as well (pulsus parvus and tardus). (See Chapter 10.)

upstroke and represents turbulence created by ejection of blood across a narrow and distorted valve orifice.

In general, the more abnormal the pulse contour and volume are, the more likely the aortic valve will be hemodynamically obstructive. *Practical Point: A rapid rate of rise and a normal pulse contour without a sustained peak usually excludes significant valvular aortic stenosis. Unfortunately, both false-positive and false-negative diagnoses occur.*

In general, children and young adults may have hemodynamically significant aortic stenosis with little detectable abnormality of the arterial pulse. In the aged, the "normal" arterial pulse often is accentuated due to a loss of distensibility of the vascular bed. The diagnostic qualities of the arterial pulse in aortic stenosis can be attenuated if there is associated systemic hypertension or aortic regurgitation. In hypertension, the rate of rise and pulse amplitude are increased in late systole. With coexisting aortic regurgitation, the large stroke volume and more rapid ejection rate may "normalize" the typical small and obstructive pulse of aortic stenosis.

The arterial pulse can simulate aortic stenosis whenever the stroke volume is reduced and a prominent systolic murmur is present, as might be found in patients with congestive heart failure, cardiomyopathy, or mitral stenosis. In such conditions, the nonspecific systolic ejection murmur may be entirely functional. In a patient with mild aortic stenosis but significantly depressed LV systolic function, the carotid pulse may suggest more severe valve obstruction than actually is present.

Table 10-2 lists the common clinical situations in which the arterial pulse can result in a false-positive or false-negative assessment of aortic stenosis.

Hypertrophic Cardiomyopathy

In hypertrophic cardiomyopathy, the early rate of rise of the arterial pulse characteristically is brisk, giving a tapping quality to the pulse. These abnormalities become more pronounced with large left ventricular-aortic gradients. However, many patients with hypertrophic cardiomyopathy have a normal carotid pulse (see Chapter 11).

Coarctation of the Aorta

In coarctation of the aorta and associated hypertension, the carotid pulses are increased in amplitude but have a normal contour. If there is associated aortic valve obstruction or stenosis due to a congenitally bicuspid aortic valve, the carotid pulse may have a slow upstroke and reduced volume. In all cases of hemodynamically significant coarctation, the femoral pulses are small in volume (occasionally impalpable) and markedly delayed with respect to simultaneous palpation of the brachial or radial pulses.

Aortic Regurgitation

In aortic regurgitation (see Chapter 12), the increased stroke volume, rapid rate of ejection, and decreased peripheral resistance result in a high-volume, bounding arterial pulse with a characteristic collapsing quality (see Figure 12-1). A systolic thrill may be present over the carotid arteries, even in the absence of aortic stenosis. With major aortic insufficiency, systolic blood pressure is increased and diastolic blood pressure is abnormally low (see Figure 12-1). The systemic arteries may appear to swell or pulsate.

The alterations in pulse wave in moderate to severe aortic regurgitation are easily detected in all peripheral arteries. In pure aortic regurgitation or mixed aortic stenosis and regurgitation, a bisferious systolic carotid pulse (double peaked) is common, suggesting hemodynamically significant aortic regurgitation (see Figure 12-2). With the onset of congestive heart failure or decreased left ventricular stroke volume, the bisferious pulse may disappear and the amplitude and pulse volume decrease. *Practical Point: The typical changes in the arterial pulse in severe aortic regurgitation may be minimal or even absent when left ventricular function is significantly depressed.*

Hyperkinetic States

Any condition associated with an increased stroke volume and decreased peripheral resistance may produce an arterial pulse that can simulate aortic regurgitation; for example, large AV fistula, thyrotoxicosis, patent ductus arteriosus, or severe anemia.

3

The Jugular Venous Pulse

Careful observation of the venous pulse can lead to valuable information about cardiac events. Examination of the neck veins often is viewed with anxiety and dismay by medical students and physicians; the terminology appears arcane, the task obscure. This chapter stresses a practical bedside approach.

Normal Physiology

Although the venous system contains about 70–80% of the circulating blood volume, it maintains a very low intravascular pressure (3–7 mmHg or 4–11 cm H_2O). Therefore, venous compliance is high; that is, veins are extremely distensible. The jugular venous pulse reflects the relationship between venous tone, the volume of blood in the venous system, and right heart hemodynamics. During diastole, the jugular veins directly reflect right ventricular filling pressure; during systole, right atrial pressure. Thus, analysis of the jugular venous pulse provides considerable information about right-sided cardiac physiology.

Waveforms

Two peaks or waves and two descents or troughs are visible in the normal jugular venous pulse (Figure 3-1). The A wave is followed by the X descent, and V wave is followed by the Y descent. When the jugular pulse or the right atrial pressure is recorded, a C wave usually is present, interrupting the X descent. The physiologic basis of these waves and descents is as follows.

A Wave

This wave directly reflects right atrial (RA) contraction, which results in retrograde blood flow into the superior vena cava and jugular veins. The jugular venous A wave follows the P wave of the EKG, precedes the upstroke of the carotid pulse, and is almost synchronous with S_1.

X Descent

The early portion of the X descent results from RA relaxation during atrial diastole. The later and dominant portion reflects the fall in right atrial pressure during early right ventricular systole, as the tricuspid valve ring is pulled caudally by the contracting right ventricle ("descent of the base").

The X descent often is the most prominent motion of the normal jugular venous pulse. It begins *during systole* and ends just before S_2.

C Wave

This positive wave has caused enormous controversy and confusion over the years. Part of the problem relates to the fact that the C wave has two different causes. In the neck veins, the C wave is an artifact caused by transmitted carotid artery pulsations; however, in the right atrium the C wave reflects the upward bulging motion of the closed tricuspid valve during isovolumic systole. *Practical Point: Because the C wave usually is not visible as a separate waveform and has no importance in the examination of the jugular venous pulse, it should be disregarded.*

V Wave

The V wave is the second major positive wave. It begins in late systole, and ends in early diastole. The V wave results from continued venous inflow into the right atrium during ventricular systole while the tricuspid valve is closed. It is roughly synchronous with the carotid pulse and peaks just after S_2.

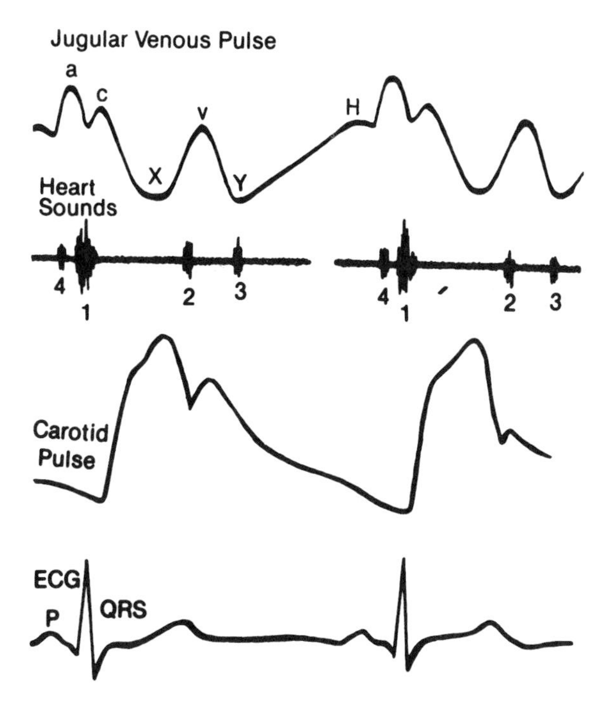

Figure 3-1. Normal jugular venous pulse. Note the biphasic venous waveform with a large A wave immediately preceding the carotid upstroke and roughly coinciding with S_1 and a smaller V wave that peaks almost coincident with S_2. The jugular X descent occurs during systole and in some individuals may be quite prominent. The Y descent occurs during early diastole; the nadir of the Y descent times with S_3. The C wave and H wave are not visible to the eye but often are recordable in venous pulse tracings.

Y Descent

The Y descent is the negative deflection of RA pressure that occurs when the tricuspid valve opens in early diastole. It begins and ends during diastole.

Practical Point: In normal persons, the right atrial A wave is larger than the V wave and the X descent is more prominent than the Y descent. When the neck veins are examined, in most conditions a larger A than V wave will be seen (see Figure 3-1).

Respiratory Influences

Inspiration may result in increased visibility of the venous pulse. During inspiration, the velocity of venous flow and the return to the right heart increases; RA and RV contraction become more vigorous (Starling effect), exaggerating the X and Y descents. Although mean venous pressure falls slightly, the waveforms are accentuated during inspiration.

The Examination

Anatomy

The venous pulse is visible but not palpable. The internal jugular vein is located in the right supraclavicular fossa between the heads of the sternocleidomastoid muscle. Usually, the internal jugular vein itself is not visible; indirect venous pulsations of the jugular bulb and internal jugular vein are transmitted to the overlying skin and soft tissues with a subtle and undulant motion that must be sought carefully. The external jugular veins, coursing vertically over the sternocleidomastoid muscle posterior and lateral to the internal jugular vein, usually are seen more easily, and the discrete venous pulsations typically are seen more easily than the internal jugular system (Figure 3-2). However, when visible, assessment of the internal jugular veins is *preferable* to the external jugular veins.

The right side of the neck is better than the left for examination of the jugular venous pulse. Nevertheless, if there is any difficulty in seeing a clearly pulsatile jugular vein on the right, *both* sides of the neck should be examined carefully.

Position of Patient

The patient should be reclining and comfortable without excessive tension on the tissues of the neck (see Figure 3-2). Often, it is helpful to elevate the chin and slightly rotate the head to the left, gently stretching the skin of the right lower neck and supraclavicular area. In hospitalized patients, removing the pillow often aids in proper positioning; however, the addition of a small pillow may be necessary for optimal visualization. Natural light is desirable for inspection of the venous pulsations, although a flashlight or bedside lamp can be used

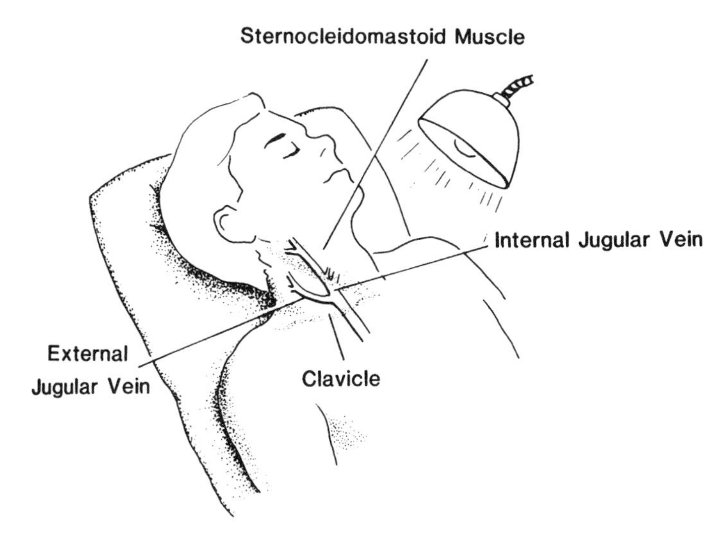

Figure 3-2. Important landmarks of the venous pulse. The external jugular veins easily are seen lateral to the sternocleidomastoid muscles, extending vertically upward toward the back of the ear. The internal jugular veins are of small amplitude and undulant in nature. They usually are not seen well in individuals with a normal venous pulse but may be prominent when the jugular venous pressure is elevated or when prominent V waves are present. The ideal patient position consists of modest elevation of the thorax and head. It is important for the patient to be relaxed with no tension on the neck muscles. Tangential lighting is helpful to accentuate the jugular veins.

profitably to cast a shadow on the venous pulsations occurring in the lower neck. For this purpose, tangential lighting is best, as it can silhouette the neck veins to great advantage.

Estimating Venous Pressure

Optimal positioning of the neck and thorax is essential for analysis of the venous pressure and waveforms. The examiner first should estimate whether the venous pressure will be normal or elevated and position the patient accordingly.

Normal Venous Pressure

In most patients without elevation of the venous pressure, the supine or 15–30° position is best. The patient's head and neck must be positioned so that the venous waveforms are clearly identifiable. During inspiration clear-cut pulsations should be visible, to ascertain that there is a patent, distortion-free venous column. The height of the venous column at the peak of the A and V waves generally is taken as an indication of the venous pressure, although the actual mean jugular venous pressure will be slightly lower.

The sternal angle (of Louis), found at the junction of the manubrium and sternum at the level of the second rib, is used as the standard reference point for determining venous pressure noninvasively. In the supine position, the right atrium is 5–7 cm below this point. Conventional wisdom has held that the right atrium is approximately 5 cm below the sternal angle at *any* body position, and therefore the height of the mean jugular venous pulse in the 30°, 45°, 60°, or 90° position was determined by measuring the distance from the angle of Louis to the estimated level of the venous column and adding to this 5 cm to give an approximation of the mean right atrial pressure. One study, however, has confirmed that this oft repeated "golden rule" is erroneous. Although, when patients are lying flat, the right atrial pressure is approximately 5 cm below the sternum, as soon as the thorax is elevated to 30° or more, the relationship between the right atrium and the sternal angle is altered such that the physician should add *10 cm* to the height of the venous column from the sternal angle to obtain an estimate of the peak venous pressure. Therefore, if the mean venous column is 3 cm above the sternal angle with the chest at 45°, the estimated venous pressure is 13 cm H_2O, which is elevated.

Using these new guidelines, one should make a diagnosis of an *elevated* mean jugular venous pressure when the thorax is positioned at 30° or greater from the horizontal and the mean peak of the venous column clearly is 2–3 cm H_2O or more above the sternal angle of Louis. In the supine position or with only a pillow under the patient's head, however, the venous column can be up to 2–3 cm above the sternal landmark and still be normal.

Elevated Venous Pressure

In conditions where the venous pressure is very high, pulsations may not be seen until the patient is sitting up; even then, the waves may be invisible. Careful inspection of the upper neck beneath the angle of the jaw is important; the external jugular veins also should be analyzed when increased levels of venous pressure are suggested. In severe tricuspid insufficiency, the ear lobes may move gently laterally with each V wave (see Figure 16-4).

Practical Point: Adequate visualization of the jugular venous pressure is difficult, if not impossible in many persons, particularly obese subjects or patients with short, thick necks. Nevertheless, with care and attention to detail, the venous pulse can be identified in the majority of subjects. Inspiration or modest elevation of the thorax frequently "brings out" the venous waveforms in patients with difficult-to-see jugular veins.

Timing of Venous Waves

Timing the venous pulse may be assessed by two methods. In the first, the left carotid pulse is carefully palpated simultaneously with visual inspection of the right-side jugular veins. In the second, the jugular venous pulse is analyzed in concert with auscultation of the heart sounds. Both techniques are useful.

Visual Technique

The first method relies on the dominance of the jugular A wave. Because RA contraction precedes LV contraction, the jugular A wave will be seen as a flickering pulsation just *before* the carotid artery pulse is felt. *Practical Point: Identification of the jugular A wave preceding the palpable carotid pulse usually is all that is necessary for accurate identification of the venous pulse waves.*

Auscultation

If present, the venous A wave is coincident with an S_4 and is approximately simultaneous with S_1. The X descent occurs during *systole* and will be seen as a negative transient occurring between S_1 and S_2, with the trough occurring just before S_2. The V wave begins in late systole and peaks just after S_2; the Y descent or collapse begins in early *diastole* after the V wave.

Hepatojugular Reflux (Abdominal Compression Test)

This technique, popularized by Ewy, employs sustained pressure applied to the right upper quadrant of the abdomen. The hepatojugular reflux test is a useful diagnostic maneuver when the jugular venous pulse is borderline elevated or when latent RV failure or silent tricuspid regurgitation is suspected. Abdominal compression forces venous blood into the thorax. A failing or dilated right ventricle may not be able to receive the augmented venous return to the right heart without a rise in mean venous pressure. In normal persons, sustained abdominal pressure will not elevate the venous pressure or will cause only a slight (1 cm) elevation that is not sustained. In congestive heart failure or tricuspid regurgitation, this maneuver will result in an elevation of the venous pressure greater than 1 cm that persists throughout the time the pressure is applied. The hepatojugular reflux test then is said to be positive (Figure 3-3).

Technique

In the abdominal compression test, the patient is positioned so that the upper level of the venous column is at mid-neck level. Gentle but firm compression of the right upper quadrant with an open-fingered hand is applied for 10–15 sec. If there is significant tenderness or discomfort over the liver, the pressure can be applied elsewhere in the abdomen with similar results.

A positive test indicates incipient or actual RV failure, pulmonary hypertension, or constructive pericarditis. In isolated LV failure, the response will be normal. Patients with hypervolemia or fluid overload will have a positive test.

Differentiation of Jugular and Carotid Pulses

Careful examination of the neck pulses, in most instances, should prevent confusing venous and carotid artery activity. In severe tricuspid regurgitation, however, venous pulsations may be palpable and visible from the foot of the bed and be confused with the arterial pulsations of severe aortic regurgitation. Table 3-1 lists the features that allow proper identification of the venous and arterial pulses in the neck.

Abnormal Variants of the Venous Pulse

Mean Pressure

Increased Mean Venous Pressure

Right ventricular failure is the most common cause of increased jugular venous pressure. Other important cardiovascular conditions

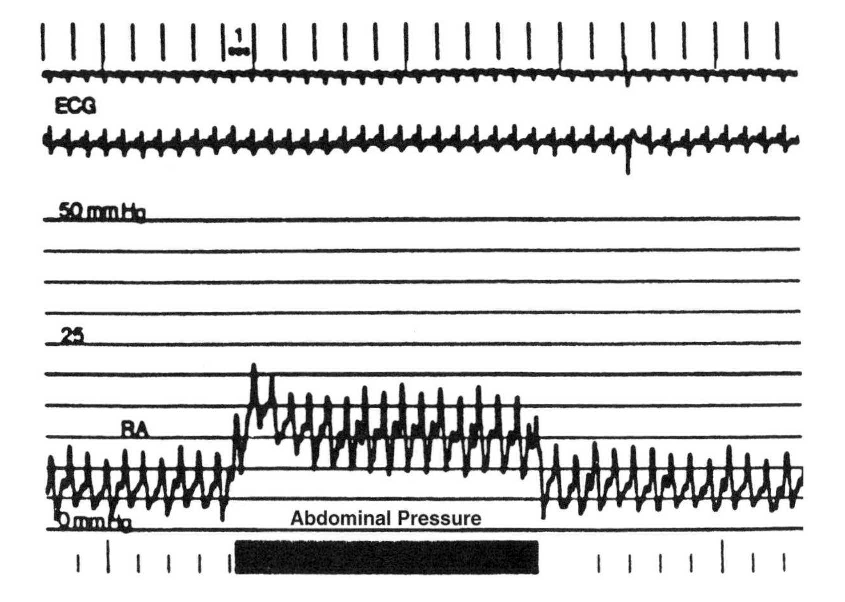

Figure 3-3. Elevation in right atrial (RA) pressure observed during abdominal pressure in patient with mild congestive heart failure. From Gordon Ewy, M.D., with permission.

associated with elevated mean venous pressure include constrictive pericarditis, pericardial tamponade, and tricuspid regurgitation due to RV hypertension. The venous pressure occasionally can be elevated in persons with a normal cardiovascular system, typically in those with a high output or hyperkinetic state. Fluid overload, obesity, or increased abdominal pressure from any cause can result in high venous pressure; and asthma, respiratory distress, and emphysema may produce distended neck veins as a result of expiratory increases in intrathoracic pressure.

RV Infarction

Recent recognition of the syndrome of right ventricular infarction has resulted in another indication for careful analysis of jugular venous pulse. Right ventricular involvement is seen in conjunction with acute inferior or diaphragmatic myocardial infarction and may manifest in

Table 3-1. Differentiation of Jugular Venous Pulsations from the Carotid Arterial Pulse

	Internal Jugular Vein	Carotid Artery
Location	Low in neck, lateral	Deep in neck, medial
Contour	Double peaked	Single peaked
Character	Undulant, not palpable	Forceful, brisk, easily felt
Inspiration	A and V waves often more visible, although mean pressure decreases	No change
Upright position	Decrease in mean pressure	No change
Compressibility	Readily obliterated by gentle pressure 3–4 cm above clavicle	Cannot compress easily
Abdominal compression	May see transient increase in pressure	No effect

a wide variety of presentations from overt shock to an isolated elevation of the venous pulse. The extension of myocardial necrosis into the adjacent right ventricle may "stiffen" the right ventricle and frequently causes an elevation of RV filling pressure. Therefore, the mean jugular venous pressure will be elevated, often with an accentuated A wave, even in the absence of an elevation of LV filling pressure. On occasion, the venous pulse in RV infarction can mimic that of constrictive pericarditis, with prominent X and Y descents producing two deep troughs in the venous pulse.

Decreased Mean Venous Pressure

Very low venous pressure may be a clue to the presence of hypovolemia or dehydration. In hypotension or overt shock, a flat or low-normal jugular venous pressure may be an invaluable clue to the underlying pathophysiology.

Increased A Wave Amplitude

Whenever the force of right atrial contraction is augmented, the A wave will increase and may become quite prominent (Figure 3-4A). When it is very large, it is known as a *giant A wave*. The most common cause of a large A wave is decreased RV compliance, usually associated with an increase in RV end-diastolic pressure. Such altered compliance is seen in RV hypertrophy from any cause, such as severe pulmonary hypertension, pulmonic stenosis, or pulmonary vascular disease.

X Descent

The systolic collapse of the jugular venous pulse becomes deeper whenever there is vigorous right ventricular contraction, as occurs in cardiac tamponade or RV overload states. The X descent also may be quite prominent in atrial septal defects. In mild tricuspid regurgitation, the X descent is attenuated and disappears with major degrees of regurgitation (Figure 3-4B).

V Wave

The classic cause of an enlarged V wave is tricuspid regurgitation (see Chapter 16), where the V wave becomes the dominant venous pulsation (see Figures 3-4B and 16-1). The V wave in tricuspid regurgitation (sometimes referred to as the CV wave or S wave) begins earlier in systole than the usual V wave and, when prominent, can simulate carotid artery pulsations. They even may be palpable. Giant V waves often are visible in the earlobes and upper neck (see Figure 16-4); these large undulant venous pulsations in the neck often can be seen from the foot of the bed.

The V wave also may increase in prominence in the setting of congestive heart failure without tricuspid regurgitation. In subjects with atrial fibrillation, the V wave can be quite large. In atrial septal defect, the V wave generally is larger than normal, and the A and V waves typically are of equal amplitude.

Y Descent

The Y descent or trough is exaggerated when the venous pressure is elevated from any cause. In constrictive pericarditis (Figure 3-4C), this prominent diastolic collapse is known as *Friedreich's sign* and usually is accompanied by a diastolic filling sound (S_3 or pericardial knock). The Y descent may be diminutive in pericardial tamponade.

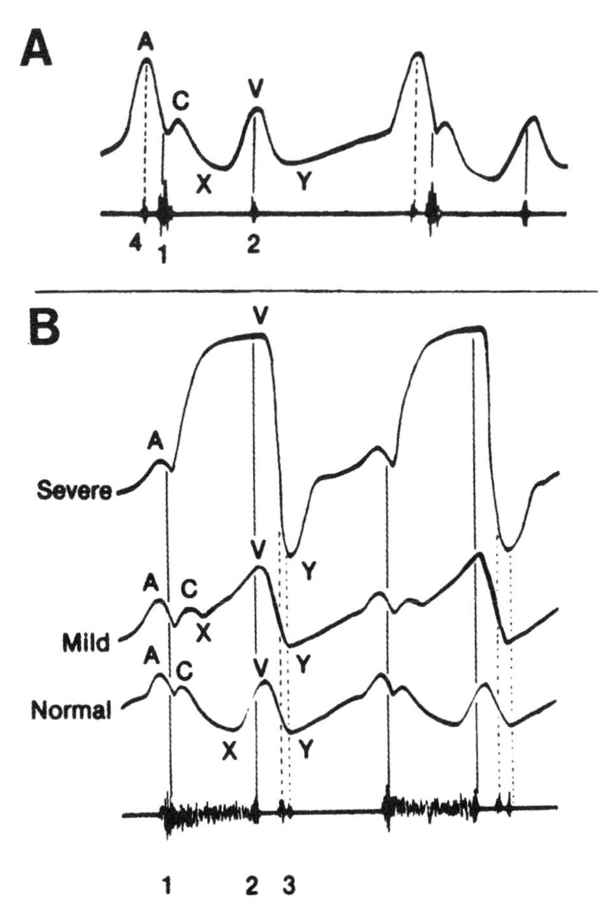

Figure 3-4. Common abnormalities of the venous pulse: (A) Large A waves associated with elevated right ventricular end-diastolic pressure or decreased right ventricular compliance. Increased A wave size or giant A waves are seen when there is severe right ventricular hypertrophy, usually associated with right ventricular systolic hypertension. A right ventricular S_4 often is present in such cases. (B) Augmented V wave in tricuspid regurgitation. As reflux across the tricuspid valve increases in severity, the systolic V wave becomes higher as well as broader. The X descent disappears and the Y descent is progressively accentuated with increasing severity of tricuspid regurgitation. With severe tricuspid regurgitation, the systolic wave may be so dominant as to mimic the carotid arterial pulsations; the entire lower neck will swell with each right ventricular systole (see Chapter 16).

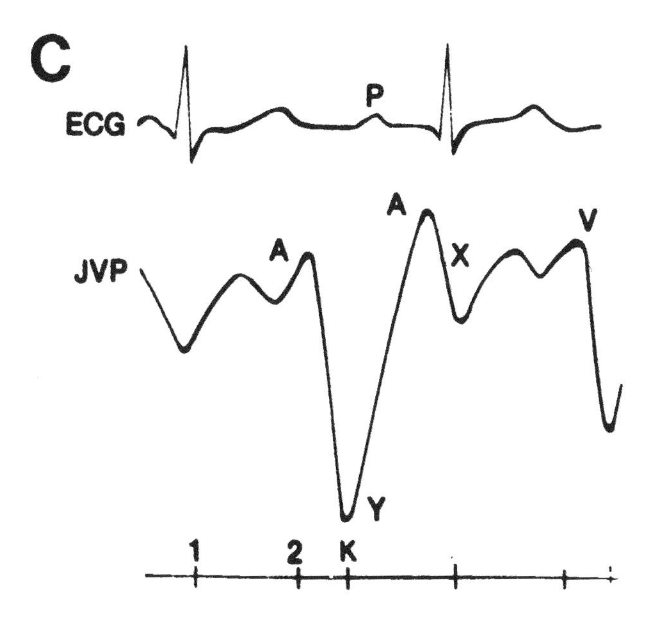

Figure 3-4. *continued* (C) Constrictive pericarditis. In this unusual cardiac condition, right ventricular diastolic pressure is greatly elevated. This elevation results in a prominent Y descent following tricuspid valve opening. The abrupt rise in venous pressure during right ventricular filling is due to the noncompliant right ventricular chamber encased in an unyielding pericardial shell. The venous pulse contour in constrictive pericarditis often takes on an *M* or *W* configuration. A pericardial knock (K), a high-frequency early diastolic filling sound, typically is present.

Inspiratory Increase in Venous Pressure (Kussmaul's Sign)

This unusual phenomenon is seen in conditions where the right ventricle has such decreased compliance or capacity that the augmented venous return occurring during inspiration cannot be adequately "handled" by the right ventricle and the venous pressure "backs up." Typically, it is seen in constrictive pericarditis (present in approximately 40% of cases) and severe congestive heart failure. It is distinctly uncommon in pericardial tamponade.

4

The Precordial Impulse

Precordial palpation enables the physician to detect cardiac activity on the chest wall. In the normal individual, cardiac motion is represented by the *apex beat* or *apex impulse,* produced by contraction of the left ventricular free wall and septum. When cardiac hypertrophy or dilatation is present, abnormal systolic and diastolic events emanating from the left or right ventricle may be detected on palpation.

Experienced clinicians can derive a great deal of information about cardiac size and function from a careful analysis of precordial motion. This chapter outlines a practical approach to precordial palpation. The focus is on *what can be felt* by the examiner.

Physiology

Normal Precordial Activity

The palpable apical impulse in a normal subject is produced by an anterior movement of the left ventricle during early systole. As isovolumic, intraventricular pressure rises, the LV rotates in a counterclockwise direction on its long axis as the cardiac apex lifts and makes contact with the left anterior chest wall. Following aortic valve opening, the LV chamber moves away from the chest wall after the first half of ejection and the ventricle continues to decrease in size until systole is completed. Therefore, the impulse felt or recorded on the precordium is comprised of an early outward thrust, followed by retraction during the last part of systole (Figure 4-1). *Practical Point: Normal palpable cardiac activity occurs only during the first half of systole.*

Peak outward motion of the apex impulse occurs coincident with or just after aortic valve opening and the beginning of ejection. The impulse is sustained for a brief period, then the outward movement ceases as the LV apex moves inward (see Figure 4-1). Diastolic events,

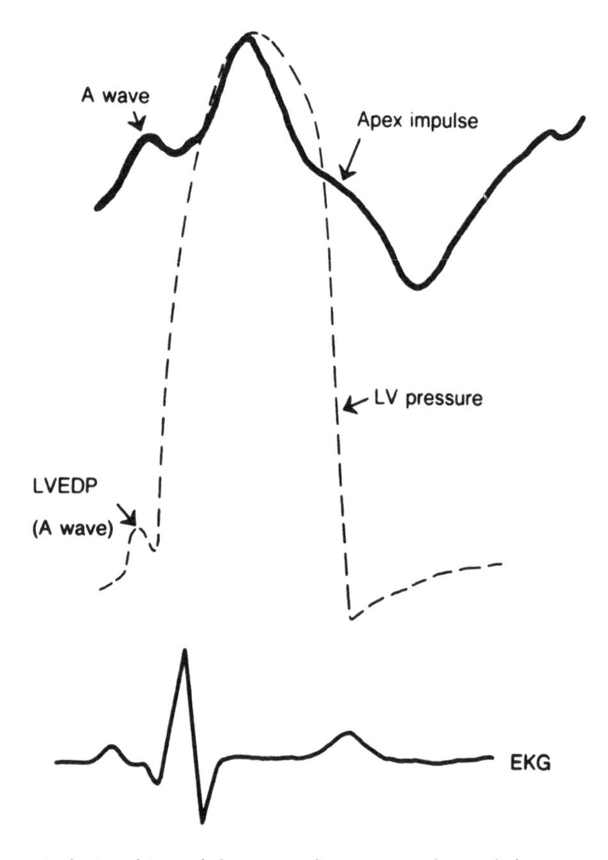

Figure 4-1. Relationships of the normal apex impulse to left ventricular pressure. LVEDP = left ventricular end-diastolic pressure. (Reprinted with permission from Abrams J. Precordial palpation. In: Horowitz LD, Groves BM, eds. *Signs and Symptoms in Cardiology.* Philadelphia: JB Lippincott Co.; 1985:157.)

such as those produced by rapid left ventricular filling (S_3) or left atrial contraction (S_4), normally are not palpable. With alterations in ventricular diastolic volume, pressure, or compliance, these events (palpable S_3 and S_4) may be felt by the examining fingers. The characteristics of the normal precordial impulse are listed in Table 4-1 and shown in Figure 4-2A.

Table 4-1. The Normal Supine Apical Impulse

- A gentle, nonsustained tap
- Early systolic anterior motion that ends before the last third of systole
- Located within 10 cm of the midsternal line in the fourth or fifth left intercostal space
- A palpable area less than 2–2.5 cm^2 and detectable in only one intercostal space
- Right ventricular motion normally not palpable
- Diastolic events normally not palpable
- May be completely absent in older persons

(Modified with permission from Abrams J. Precordial palpation. In: Horowitz LD, Groves BM, eds. *Signs and Symptoms in Cardiology.* Philadelphia: JB Lippincott Co.; 1985:167.)

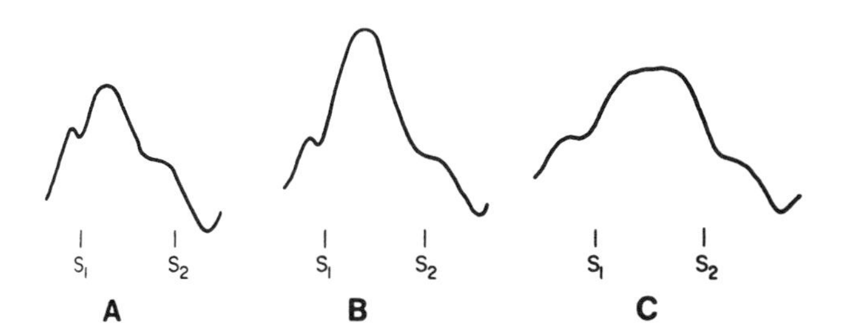

Figure 4-2. Major types of left ventricular precordial motion: (A) normal; (B) hyperdynamic; (C) sustained. With a patient in the supine position, the presence of sustained left ventricular activity detectable in the latter half of systole is distinctly abnormal. Some experts believe that palpation of a sustained impulse when patients are in the left lateral decubitus position may have less specificity for underlying left ventricular enlargement. (Reprinted with permission from Abrams J. Precordial palpation. In: Horowitz LD, Groves BM, eds. *Signs and Symptoms in Cardiology.* Philadelphia: JB Lippincott Co.; 1985:158.)

Right Ventricular Activity

Although the right ventricle, located just beneath the sternum and left third to fifth ribs, is closer to the chest wall than the left ventricle, RV activity normally is not felt. In normal children and young adults or thin subjects who have a narrow AP thoracic diameter, gentle right ventricular activity occasionally may be felt.

Abnormalities of Precordial Motion

When there are abnormalities in ventricular size, shape, or function, precordial activity is detected more easily (Tables 4-2 and 4-3). The left and right ventricular precordial impulse may be altered in *location, amplitude, size,* or *contour.* Almost all diagnostic alterations in precordial motion occur in systole. Table 4-3 summarizes the most common abnormalities of the apical impulse.

Systolic Events

Left Ventricle

Characteristic changes may occur in the apical impulse with LV enlargement, depending on whether hypertrophy or dilatation is dominant. Such abnormalities often provide the clinician with the first clue of organic heart disease. Left ventricular wall motion abnormalities, focal or generalized, frequently are manifest by an abnormal apex motion pattern.

Table 4-2. Causes of Palpable Precordial Abnormalities

LV hypertrophy or dilatation
LV wall motion abnormalities (fixed or transient)
Increased force of left atrial contraction (palpable S_4)
Accentuated diastolic rapid filling (palpable S_3)
Anterior thrust of the heart from severe mitral regurgitation
RV hypertrophy or dilatation
Loud murmurs (thrills)
Loud heart sounds (normal and abnormal)
Dilated or hyperkinetic pulmonary artery
Dilated aorta

Table 4-3. Major Types of Precordial Impulses

	Hyperkinetic	Sustained	Late Systolic
Left ventricular impulse (apex beat)	Hyperkinetic circulatory states Thin chest wall Pectus excavatum Volume overload: Aortic regurgitation Mitral regurgitation Ventricular septal defect	Pressure overload: Hypertension Aortic stenosis Chronic or severe volume overload states LV dilatation, especially with decreased ejection fraction LV dysfunction LV aneurysm	LV dyssynergy Hypertrophic cardiomyopathy Mitral valve prolapse (rare)
Right ventricular impulse (parasternal area)	Hyperkinetic circulatory state in young subjects Volume overload: Atrial septal defect Tricuspid regurgitation	Pressure overload: Pulmonary stenosis Pulmonary hypertension Cor pulmonale Mitral stenosis Pulmonary emboli Cardiomyopathy	Severe mitral regurgitation

(Reprinted with permission from Abrams J. Precordial motion in health and disease. *Mod Con Cardiovasc Dis*. 1980;49:55–60.)

Volume Overload The classic response to significant volume overload conditions is an *increase in the amplitude* (hyperkinetic impulse) of the LV impulse with no change in contour: Early systolic outward and late systolic inward motion is preserved. Early or mild degrees of mitral or aortic regurgitation, classic overload states, may not alter the amplitude or contour of the LV impulse. In severe volume overload, particularly with depression of LV contractility and a decreased ejection fraction, the LV impulse may become *prolonged* or *sustained* into the second half of systole. With cardiac dilatation, the normal elliptical LV shape becomes more spherical and the resulting apical impulse becomes sustained. Left ventricular dilatation with a major increase in LV end-diastolic volume also results in *leftward and downward displacement* of the apex impulse, as well as an *increase in the size* of the actual contact area of the apex beat.

Pressure Overload The initial response of the LV to increased outflow resistance (aortic stenosis, hypertension) is concentric hypertrophy with no increase in cavity size. Systolic function is well maintained. With time, the LV impulse becomes *prolonged* in duration, reflecting an increased left ventricular ejection time. This produces a sustained left ventricular heave or thrust. The force of contraction is increased, but there is relatively little chamber dilatation. Therefore, the apex impulse usually is not displaced but has an *increased force*. With long-standing disease and depression of cardiac function, the LV chamber dilates and the impulse moves more laterally on the chest wall. The apex beat in pressure-loaded hearts usually is not felt over as large an area of the chest wall, like that in chronic severe volume overload states.

Abnormalities of Left Ventricular Systolic Function When LV contractile performance is deranged, the apical impulse can be altered in several ways:

1. The normal brief outward contour may become sustained into the last half of systole, which may result from ischemic dysfunction due either to fibrosis or to depressed myocardial contractile performance or from LV dilatation and a globally depressed ejection fraction.
2. A mid- or late-systolic impulse (bulge) may be present, reflecting a disordered contraction pattern (coronary heart disease or cardiomyopathy).

3. An ectopic precordial impulse may appear, located at a site away from the normal apical impulse, usually superior and medial to it, which is most likely to occur with an LV aneurysm but may be seen with anterior wall dyskinesis in the absence of an overt aneurysm.
4. Inferolateral displacement and enlargement of the area of the apex beat will be present whenever the LV chamber is substantially dilated, particularly if there is a depressed ejection fraction.

Hyperdynamic States Anxiety, tachycardia, exertion, or catechol excess from any cause may increase cardiac contractility and systolic blood pressure, resulting in an increase in the force and amplitude of the apex impulse. In such situations, the location and contour of the precordial impulse is unchanged; the apex impulse increases in forcefulness but is not sustained (hyperkinetic) (see Figure 4-2B).

Right Ventricle
The right ventricle responds similarly to the LV with respect to volume and pressure overload states.

Volume Overload The volume-loaded RV (atrial septal defect, tricuspid regurgitation without RV dysfunction) produces a hyperdynamic, high-amplitude impulse that retains the pattern of mid–late systolic retraction. Therefore, the motion is a brief anterior thrust. With a very large RV end-diastolic volume or depressed RV contractile function, this anterior parasternal motion may become sustained.

Pressure Overload Pulmonary hypertension from any cause results in sustained systolic RV activity manifest as a palpable or visible anterior motion in the lower left sternal area (see Figure 13-3C).

Diastolic Events

Left Ventricle
Left ventricular diastolic filling comprises two phases: initial rapid filling following mitral valve opening and late diastolic augmentation resulting from left atrial contraction (see Figure 6-1). In the normal heart, these filling events (and their resultant heart sounds) are neither palpable nor audible.

When ischemia, fibrosis, hypertrophy, or dilatation is present, LV compliance, diastolic volume, and filling pressure are altered so that the two peaks of blood flow from the left atrium to the LV may result in large pressure transients and increased distending forces. *In these situations, the rapid filling phase and left atrial systole may result in audible and palpable events (S_3 and S_4).*

Palpable S_3 An abnormal increase in transmitral flow, a large LV end-diastolic volume, and significant depression of LV function all are associated with the presence of an audible S_3, which may be palpable. A palpable S_3 commonly is found in patients with a major elevation in LV filling pressure and LV end-diastolic volume. Typically, these hearts have a decreased ejection fraction. Patients with aortic valve disease, hypertensive heart disease, or coronary heart disease may develop a loud or palpable S_3 when LV systolic function deteriorates. Patients with congestive cardiomyopathy often have a palpable LV filling sound. The pericardial knock of constrictive pericarditis is an early, exaggerated filling event, comparable to a loud S_3, and usually is palpable.

In subjects with an increased volume and rate of blood flow crossing the mitral valve, an S_3 may be audible and palpable *in the presence of good left ventricular function.* Classically, severe mitral regurgitation is the cause of such filling events: A voluminous amount of blood returns to the LV from the left atrium during the rapid filling phase.

Palpable S_4 A palpable S_4 is related to decreased LV compliance, usually a result of hypertrophy without dilatation or ischemia with increased diastolic stiffness. *A palpable S_4 always is associated with an elevated LV end-diastolic pressure.* It commonly is found in aortic valve disease, hypertrophic cardiomyopathy, hypertensive heart disease, coronary artery disease, and occasional congestive cardiomyopathy.

Other Causes of Palpable Cardiovascular Activity

In addition to the tactile precordial phenomena related to LV and RV systolic and diastolic events, palpable precordial activity occasionally is detectable as a result of vascular pulsations or ectopic left ventricular wall motion abnormalities (see Table 4-2).

Aorta

A palpable aortic impulse never is a normal finding. When the ascending aorta or aortic arch is enlarged or dilated, palpable systolic pulsations may be detected. Therefore, with aortic aneurysms, diffuse aortic dilatation, or aortic dissection a systolic impulse may be felt in the right first or second intercostal space, the right or left sternoclavicular junction, or in the suprasternal area. A tracheal tug may be present with a large ascending aortic aneurysm. Dilatation and tortuosity of the brachiocephalic vessels also may cause prominent vascular pulsations at the suprasternal notch or above the clavicles.

Pulmonary Artery
Dilatation or enlargement of the pulmonary artery usually is associated with pulmonary hypertension, causing a palpable systolic impulse in the second–third left interspace, just to the left of the sternal edge. This is easily detectable in thin subjects.

Left Ventricular Ectopic Impulse
Focal wall motion abnormalities or an overt left ventricular aneurysm may produce systolic impulses that are detectable at sites away from the LV apex beat, usually medial and superior to the apical area. With anteroseptal scarring or dyskinesis, the ectopic impulse may be found at the lower parasternal edge and so may simulate right ventricular activity.

Palpable Heart Sound and Murmurs
Loud sound transients, such as an increased S_1, A_2, or P_2, often are palpable; these are known as *precordial shocks*. The opening snap and loud S_1 of mitral stenosis commonly are palpable, and on occasion, an alert physician can diagnose this valve lesion by palpation prior to using the stethoscope. A palpable S_2 at the second left interspace suggests systemic or pulmonary hypertension. Ejection clicks may be felt easily; the aortic ejection sound is detected at the left ventricular apex, and a pulmonic ejection sound is palpable at the upper left sternal border.

Thrills
Any loud murmur may be transmitted to the chest wall and produce a vibratory sensation detectable by the examining hand. These palpable murmurs or thrills correlate with a murmur intensity of grade 4/6 or greater. In thin subjects, the likelihood of a thrill is greater than in muscular or fleshy patients. A diastolic thrill occasionally may be felt at the apex in the lateral decubitus position in mitral stenosis or at the lower left sternal border in acute aortic regurgitation secondary to a perforated or ruptured aortic cusp.

Clinical Presentation

Examination of the Precordium

For optimal precordial examination, it is important for the examiner and subject to be relaxed and the patient's chest have maximum exposure. The room should be comfortably warm. Clothing and undergarments must be removed to allow unobstructed visualization and palpation of the chest.

The subject should be lying comfortably in a supine position or with the thorax elevated no more than 30° (Figure 4-3). *Practical Point: Patients with suspect or definite cardiovascular disease routinely should be examined both in the supine and left lateral decubitus positions; the subject should be instructed to turn on his or her left side at a 45–60° angle with the examining table and elevate the left arm over the head so that the physician may have unobstructed access to the left precordium* (Figure 4-4).

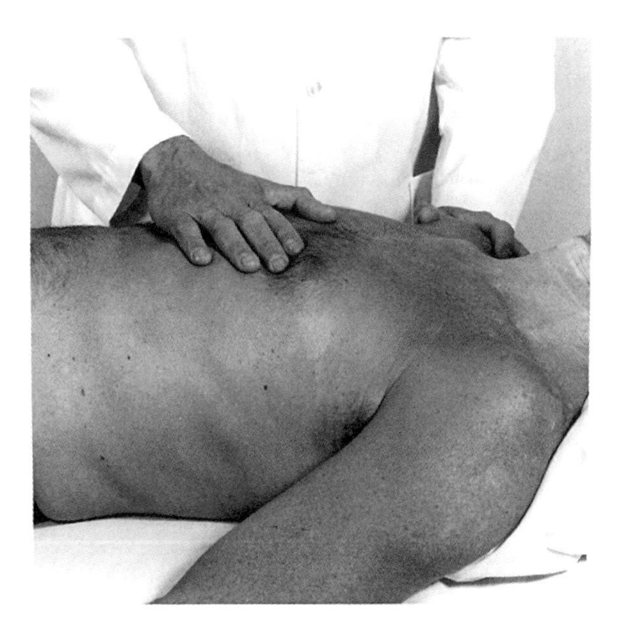

Figure 4-3. Palpation of the apex, supine position.

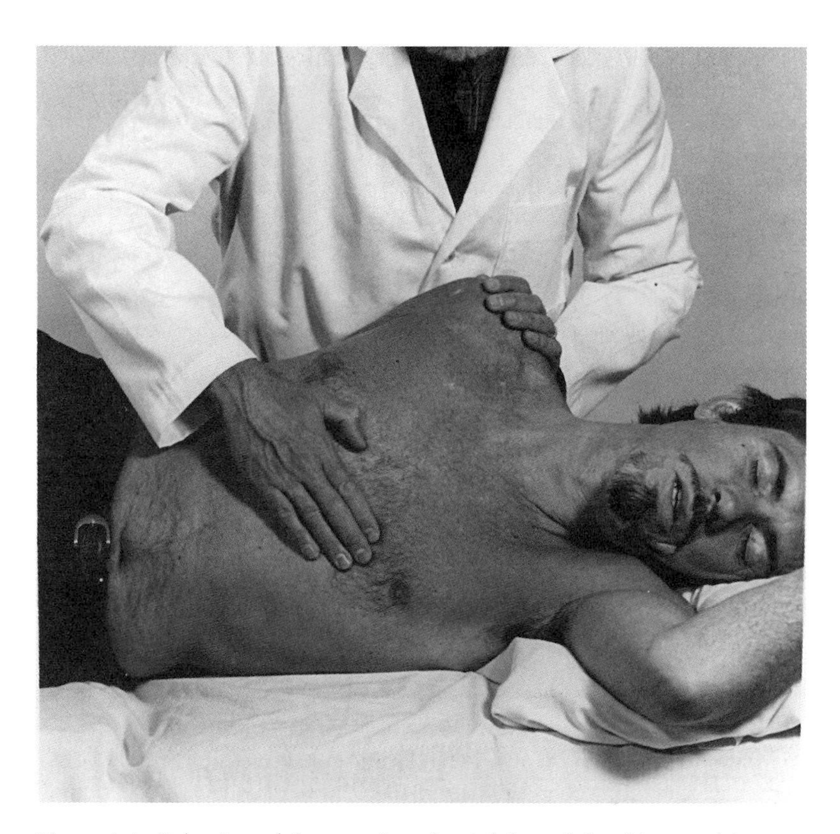

Figure 4-4. Palpation of the apex impulse, left lateral decubitus position. This maneuver should be used in any patient with suspected left ventricular disease. The patient should be turned 45–60° onto the left side with the left arm extended above the head. (Reprinted with permission from Abrams J. Precordial palpation. In: Horowitz LD, Groves BM, eds. *Signs and Symptoms in Cardiology.* Philadelphia: JB Lippincott Co.; 1985:165.)

Inspection

Careful visual observation of the chest is useful in the precordial examination; this may be more helpful after preliminary palpation has identified the site of the apex beat or other impulses, if present. Retraction movements may be more obvious to the eye than outward motion and can be quite prominent with severe degrees of left and right ventricular enlargement. Tangential lighting with the examining lamp or a penlight may accentuate visible movements on the chest wall.

Normal persons may show a slight retraction of the thorax medial to the apex impulse. As the LV thrust becomes more vigorous (hyperdynamic states, left ventricular enlargement), this retraction becomes accentuated and assumes a rocking character.

Pulmonary artery lifts commonly are visible, as may be an accentuated LV rapid ventricular filling wave (S_3), which often is more easily seen than felt.

Palpation

The examiner should be standing comfortably at the patient's right side. Both the palm of the hand and the ventral surface of the proximal metacarpals and fingers may be used for palpation. One should focus on which aspect of the hand is best for optimal tactile perception.

Varying pressure should be applied once the precordial impulse is identified. High-frequency sounds, such as an increased S_1, opening snap, or transmitted thrill, are best detected with firm application of the hand to the chest. However, the subtle low-frequency motion of a palpable S_3 or S_4 or double systolic apical impulse will be felt only with light pressure of the fingers and may be totally obscured if this examination is not performed correctly. If there is abundant precordial musculature or adipose tissue, it often is necessary to press quite firmly.

The timing of precordial events is best carried out using simultaneous palpation of the carotid arterial pulse with the left hand. Some find that concomitant auscultation of S_1 and S_2 is useful for timing purposes.

Right Ventricle

It is desirable to use held end expiration for the right ventricular examination. Firm pressure using the palm or heel of the hand with the wrist cocked upward is advisable (Figure 4-5; see also Figure 14-3B). The lower sternum and adjacent third through fifth ribs and left interspaces should be examined in this manner. *Movement of the examining hand and fingers should be carefully sought, as the typical low amplitude RV activity often is better seen than felt.*

Some experts also suggest exploring the subxyphoid or epigastric region with the extended fingers oriented superiorly; the patient should be instructed to hold his or her breath in end inspiration as the descending right ventricle is carefully palpated. This technique is particularly useful in patients with an increased AP diameter, COPD, obesity, or muscular chest when right ventricular enlargement is suspected but a parasternal impulse cannot be felt.

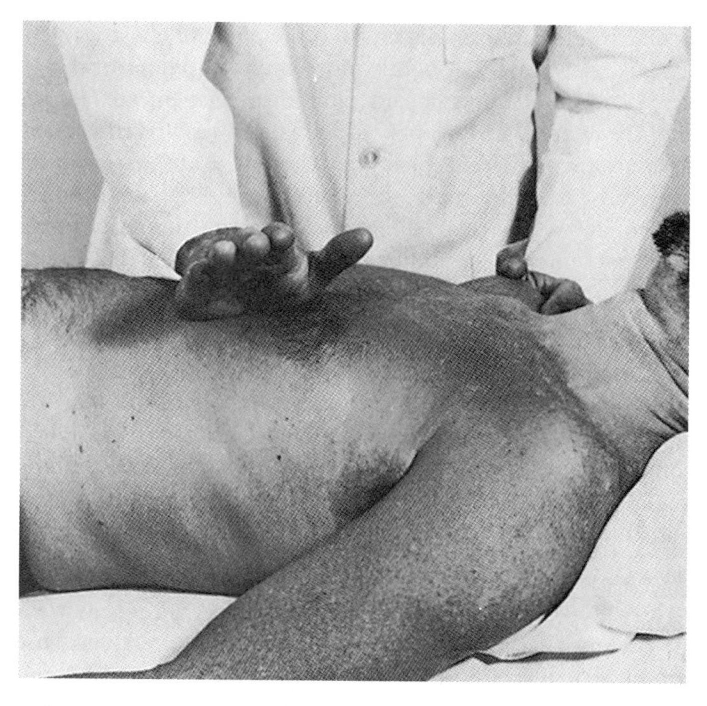

Figure 4-5. Precordial palpation for detection of parasternal or right ventricular activity. Use firm downward pressure with the heel of the hand while the patient's breath is held in end expiration.

Characteristics of the Normal Apex Impulse

In normal subjects, the apex impulse in the supine position or at a 30° elevation produces a gentle outward motion that usually is felt in only one interspace (see Table 4-1). This anterior movement is brief and nonsustained, pulling away from the examining fingers by midsystole. It occupies a maximal area of 2–2.5 cm (no larger than a quarter) and is found in the fourth or fifth left interspace at or inside the midclavicular line. It usually is found within 7–8 cm from the left sternal edge and should not be located more than 10 cm to the left of the midsternal line. In tall, thin persons, the apex beat can be distal (sixth interspace) and more medial than usual; when there is intrathoracic disease or a short stocky body habitus, the apex beat may be displaced leftward. There may be respiratory alteration in the amplitude of the apical beat; pay attention to end expiration if the impulse is hard to locate, although peak amplitude occasionally may occur during early inspiration.

In the left lateral decubitus position the point of chest wall contact of the apex beat usually is slightly more lateral and inferior than in the supine position. There is considerable disagreement centers around whether the contour of the apex impulse becomes altered when a subject assumes the left lateral position. A recent study suggested that an apical impulse of 3 cm in area or greater in the left lateral position is specific for left ventricular enlargement. In the supine position, the palpable apex impulse should be no larger than a nickel (2–3 cm) and felt in only one intercostal space.

Right Ventricular Activity

In the normal subject, parasternal activity usually is not detectable except in young or thin persons. In such cases, a gentle shock or tap at the lower left sternal border may be felt. Forceful, sustained, or high amplitude parasternal motion always is an abnormal finding (see Figure 13-3C). Occasionally a pulmonary artery impulse in the second–third left interspace adjacent to the sternum may be detected.

Point of Maximum Impulse

Many textbooks and articles in the literature use the acronym PMI to denote the apex beat. Although not ideal, this expression is used so commonly that it has become acceptable. Nevertheless, it should be recognized that *PMI* and *apical impulse* may not necessarily be synonymous.

Other Palpable Events

In a subject with suspected cardiac disease, the examiner should explore the entire precordium with firm pressure of the hand and proximal fingers, analyzing the aortic, pulmonic, lower sternal, and apical regions. In such a fashion, the unexpected vascular impulse, such as a dilated or aneurysmal ascending aorta or pulmonary artery, may be detected. Particular attention should be given to the upper sternal area, manubrium, and adjacent first and second interspaces below the medial aspect of the clavicles. Aortic pulsations and systolic thrills often are found here.

If a patient has coronary artery disease, particularly previous myocardial infarction, careful examination for an ectopic impulse should be carried out. This typically occurs medial and superior to the apex impulse. The use of the entire palm and proximal metacarpals will help detect the diffuse lift of a very large left or right ventricle; on occasion, the entire anterior precordium will move in systole. This technique also is suited for the detection of thrills and palpable heart sounds.

Percussion

Under ordinary circumstances, percussion is not a useful and necessary procedure. When a PMI cannot be identified in the supine position, this technique may help establish the presence or absence of cardiomegaly and help identify the approximate left border of the heart.

Variation of the Apex Beat: Absent Apical Impulse

It is not commonly realized that many older subjects (over age 50) have no palpable cardiac activity when examined in the supine position. This may be due to an age-related increase in the AP thoracic diameter, an increase of muscle or fat on the chest wall, or a physiologic decrease in the force of LV contraction with age. Whenever an apical impulse cannot be felt in the supine position, the left heart border should be percussed, and the patient should be carefully examined in the left lateral decubitus position (see Figure 4-4). The latter is a much more valuable maneuver than percussion. In most adults, LV activity can be detected when the subject is turned onto the left side, particularly in expiration; often the PMI becomes identifiable after the patient is again turned supine. In some normal adults, an apex impulse will not be detectable in either position.

What to Look For

The assessment of the apical cardiac impulse should include analysis of the following parameters: location, duration, size, force, and contour. In addition, visual inspection of the chest for the presence of prominent retraction waves, as well as systolic and diastolic events, should be carried out. As already mentioned, a complete precordial examination consists of a systematic evaluation of the lower sternal area, pulmonary and aortic regions, and sternoclavicular sites.

Characteristics of the Apex Impulse

Location

Identify the site of impulse on the thorax with respect to both the longitudinal and horizontal axes of the patient. Note in which intercostal space the PMI or apex beat is located; occasionally, a large heart will result in detectable precordial activity in two or even three intercostal spaces. Localize the apical impulse with reference to the midclavicular line, distance from the midsternum, or relationship to the left anterior axillary line.

Duration

The duration of the systolic outward motion probably is the most important feature of the precordial examination. *Practical Point: Although cardiomegaly or hypertrophy can exist in the presence of a brief "normal" outward movement, or even when the PMI is absent, a truly sustained left ventricular impulse in the supine or 30° elevation position is distinctly abnormal* (Figure 4-2C). Such findings suggest a pressure-overloaded ventricle (e.g., aortic stenosis, hypertension), a depressed LV ejection fraction, or a substantially dilated LV cavity.

The critical point to assess is whether or not the impulse "stays up" into the second half of systole. Proper timing of the apex beat using simultaneous auscultation of S_1 and S_2 is essential in making this observation. With practice, one can be quite accurate in assessing the actual duration of the apex impulse. Simple observation of movement of the head of the stethoscope resting on the PMI may be helpful.

Left Lateral Decubitus Position

It is unclear whether an LV impulse that becomes sustained when the patient is turned into the left lateral position (see Figures 4-4 and 6-3) but is of normal duration in the supine position has the same specificity for left ventricular enlargement as a sustained impulse or LV heave present when the patient is lying flat. In general, a definite *sustained* impulse in the left lateral position is suggestive of true LV dilatation. False positives may occur, however, and echocardiography is recommended in equivocal cases.

Size

If the apex impulse is larger than normal, it is useful to note the area of contact with the chest. Any impulse greater than 2–2.5 cm in the supine position or more than 3 cm in the left decubitus position represents cardiac enlargement.

Force or Amplitude

Is the apex beat a soft, unimpressive impulse or does it lift the examining fingers off the chest wall? Is the anterior or outward excursion greater than normal, consistent with a hyperdynamic or hyperkinetic PMI? An increase in force is consistent with LV hypertrophy and preserved systolic function. Assessment of the force of contraction is the most subjective and least quantifiable aspect of precordial examination.

Contour

The normal apical impulse consists of a brief, nonsustained anterior motion in early systole (see Figure 4-1). A sustained LV beat is the commonest abnormality of contour, but occasionally other patterns are noted.

A double systolic impulse may be seen in hypertrophic obstructive cardiomyopathy and occasionally in some patients with severe left ventricular dyssynergy or an LV aneurysm in coronary artery disease. Presystolic distention commonly is found in the left lateral position in patients who have decreased LV compliance, such as coronary artery disease, hypertensive heart disease, or aortic valve disease (see Figure 6-2 and later in this chapter).

Palpable A Wave (Presystolic Distention)

A palpable A wave usually is detected in the left decubitus position. The apex beat is carefully identified, and varying pressure with the pads of the fingers is applied at the site of the LV impulse. A double, early systolic impulse is noted, which feels like a "shelf" or ridge on the upstroke of the beat (see Figure 6-2). Usually lighter pressure will maximize tactile perception of this low amplitude finding, whereas firm pressure with the fingers may make it more difficult or impossible to feel. On occasion, presystolic distention can be prominent.

The palpable A wave reflects a high LV end-diastolic pressure and decreased LV compliance. It is an important observation as it documents a definite abnormality and suggests the presence of LV hypertrophy and increased chamber stiffness (Table 4-4). Audibility of the S_4 does not correlate with palpability; presystolic distention may be detectable when the S_4 is quite soft. Occasionally, one is unable to hear an S_4, although it is clearly palpable.

Table 4-4. Causes of a Palpable A Wave (Presystolic Distention)

- Aortic stenosis
- Hypertrophic cardiomyopathy (IHSS)
- Coronary artery disease, acute and chronic
- Acute mitral regurgitation
- Aortic regurgitation (severe or acute)
- Long-standing hypertension

Palpable S_3

The third sound often is less palpable than an S_4. It most often is found in severe mitral regurgitation or a markedly dilated cardiomyopathic ventricle. As with the S_4, palpation of the LV S_3 is greatly enhanced in the left decubitus position. The S_3 will be noted as a brief outward motion occurring in early diastole that gently taps the examiner's finger pads.

Parasternal or Right Ventricular Impulses

All of the preceding also applies to the evaluation of RV or parasternal activity. However, the low-amplitude impulse produced by right ventricular hypertrophy or dilatation usually is more difficult to evaluate than left ventricular apical activity. Nevertheless, an increase in amplitude or sustained parasternal motion usually is discernible with careful examination technique.

Right ventricular abnormalities are detectable only in the supine position. Firm downward pressure with the hand on the lower left sternal area usually is necessary; the patient should be alerted that the examiner will be pushing down on the sternum (see Figure 4-5). Since RV activity usually is of low amplitude, it will not be detected without such firm compression. Held end expiration may be very useful in detecting a subtle or slight RV lift.

In adults with RV enlargement from acquired heart disease, pulmonary hypertension invariably is present. A palpable P_2 and pulmonary artery impulse in the second or third interspace should be sought in these patients to provide valuable confirmatory evidence for RV hypertrophy.

Precordial Motion Abnormalities in Specific Cardiovascular Disorders

This section summarizes the major palpable findings in a variety of common adult cardiovascular conditions (see Table 4-3).

Aortic Stenosis

In mild aortic stenosis, the PMI may be normal. The apical impulse in hemodynamically significant valvular aortic stenosis is sustained, with outward motion remaining palpable in late systole (see Figures 4-2C and 10-4, also Chapter 10). The impulse typically is forceful and readily displaces the examining fingers. Unless LV function is impaired or LV dilatation has occurred, the apical impulse usually is not displaced laterally more than 1–2 cm from the normal location.

The impulse may be felt in more than one interspace in severe aortic stenosis. Presystolic distention of the LV (palpable A wave) is common in such situations, particularly in the left lateral position (see Figures 6-2 and 10-4). *Practical Point: A palpable S_4 in a patient with aortic stenosis correlates with a large left ventricular-aortic pressure gradient (unless there is coexisting coronary or hypertensive heart disease).*

A systolic thrill at the second right interspace often is present in valvular aortic stenosis. In older patients or those with an increased thoracic diameter, a systolic thrill occasionally is detected at the apex. An aortic stenosis thrill usually is best felt with the subject upright and leaning forward while holding the breath at end-expiration.

Aortic Regurgitation

In mild to moderate aortic regurgitation (see Chapter 12), the apex impulse may not be displaced but typically will be hyperdynamic and unsustained (Figure 4-2B). As the left ventricular cavity enlarges, the PMI is displaced laterally and downward and often takes up two or more interspaces. With major volume overload secondary to aortic regurgitation, a sustained apical impulse often is present, indicating severe LV cavity dilatation. In the left lateral position, presystolic distention (palpable S_4) may be felt. An audible or palpable S_4 excludes coexisting mitral stenosis, often suggested by the presence of a diastolic rumbling murmur known as the Austin Flint murmur (see Chapters 12 and 14).

Mitral Regurgitation

The apex impulse is normal to hyperdynamic in mild to moderate mitral regurgitation (see Chapter 13). In severe mitral regurgitation, particularly when chronic, the LV impulse is displaced laterally and has an increased force and amplitude. If the PMI is sustained, this suggests that LV systolic function has decreased and the ejection fraction is abnormal or that major LV dilatation has occurred. The apical impulse may be quite large and detectable in two or more interspaces. It is common to feel a systolic apical thrill in severe mitral regurgitation.

Mitral regurgitation may produce a *late* systolic impulse at the parasternal area or lower left sternal border (see Figure 13-3). This outward motion can be quite prominent, reflecting the systolic jet of a large volume of blood into a dilated left atrium that expands during LV ejection (see Figure 13-4). If there is coexisting pulmonary hypertension, the parasternal impulse will be sustained throughout systole.

Mitral Stenosis

In mitral stenosis (see Chapter 14), S_1 typically is palpable at the apex or medially. S_2 may be palpable if there is pulmonary hypertension (increased P_2). The opening snap commonly is palpable between the lower left sternal border and apex, especially in thin persons. In the left lateral position, a diastolic thrill may be manifest at the apex but usually is palpable only over a small area.

Left ventricular activity in pure mitral stenosis is unimpressive. However, most patients with moderate to severe degrees of mitral stenosis will have a parasternal or right ventricular lift. The more vigorous and sustained is the right ventricular lift, the more likely significant pulmonary hypertension will be present.

Hypertrophic Cardiomyopathy

In the unusual condition of hypertrophic cardiomyopathy (IHSS; see Chapter 11), precordial palpation may be quite informative. Left ventricular compliance is markedly decreased. Therefore, the A wave typically is very prominent and usually palpable and the left ventricular impulse is forceful and vigorous. The heart usually is not displaced to the left. A mid- or late-systolic secondary "bulge" may be present, resulting in a double or bifid precordial impulse (see Figure 11-2).

A systolic thrill, usually somewhat superior and medial to the apex, often is present. The murmur and thrill in hypertrophic cardiomyopathy typically do not radiate to the neck, in contradistinction to aortic stenosis.

Cardiomyopathy

The typical precordial finding in congestive cardiomyopathy is a diffuse anterior precordial motion; it often is difficult to be sure that this originates entirely from the left ventricle. The LV impulse is sustained and displaced inferolaterally, may or may not be forceful, and usually occupies more than one interspace. Presystolic distention (palpable A wave) and a palpable S_3 are common. Parasternal activity often is present; this contributes to the diffuse heaving or rocking precordial motion typical in such patients.

Coronary Artery Disease

In patients with angina pectoris who have no history of myocardial infarction, the apical impulse usually is normal, although presystolic distention occasionally may be noted in the left lateral position (see Figure 6-2). A palpable S_4 probably is the most common abnormality of precordial motion in subjects with coronary artery disease. It is important to examine all patients with suspected or proven coronary artery disease in the left lateral decubitus position for optimal palpation and auscultation.

In subjects with prior myocardial infarction the apical impulse may be normal, sustained, or ectopic or there may be late systolic motion suggesting LV dyssynergy. Ectopic impulses are common in patients with left ventricular aneurysms or severe LV dyssynergy. If there is anteroseptal dyssynergy, a parasternal lift may be present, simulating right ventricular hypertrophy. A sustained apex impulse suggests either LV hypertrophy or a wall motion abnormality.

5

The First and Second Heart Sounds

First Heart Sound (S_1)

In general, abnormalities of S_1 do not provide many important clues in cardiac physical diagnosis. Alteration in intensity of S_1 is the most useful observation that can aid the clinician.

Normal Physiology

The first heart sound (S_1) signals the onset of left ventricular contraction. Pressure within the LV begins to develop just prior to S_1 (see Figure 1-1). Left ventricular pressure rises above LA pressure well *before* the forward flow across the mitral valve ceases and the valve leaflets have reached their maximally closed position.

Two major, medium–high-frequency components of S_1 usually can be heard in normal people ("split S_1"). The first major component of S_1 (M_1) is coincident with the maximal closing excursion of the mitral cusps. Echophonocardiograms have confirmed the coincidence of tricuspid valve closure (T_1) with the second component of S_1.

Factors Affecting Intensity of S_1

PR Interval

A shorter PR interval results in late mitral valve closure and a loud S_1 (Table 5-1). When the PR is short, left ventricular pressure is higher at the time of LV-LA pressure crossover, causing a more rapid mitral valve closing motion and an increased intensity of S_1. The relative distance between the two mitral valve leaflets at the beginning of mechanical systole also is important. If the mitral valve already has closed or the leaflets are closing, the first sound is soft; if the leaflets remain open deep within the LV at the onset of systole, S_1 is loud.

Maximal (increased) intensity of S_1 occurs at a PR interval range of 80–140 msec. PR intervals over 140 msec (0.15 sec) result in a normal S_1, and PR intervals greater than 200 msec produce an attenuated or absent S_1 because the mitral valve has closed prior to development of LV pressure.

Left Ventricular Contractility

In general, the more vigorous is the LV contraction, the louder the S_1. Depressed LV contractility will result in an S_1 of decreased intensity.

Table 5-1. Factors Affecting the Intensity of S_1

Loud S_1
Short PR interval (<160 msec)
Tachycardia or hyperkinetic states
"Stiff" left ventricle
Mitral stenosis
Left atrial myxoma
Holosystolic mitral valve prolapse
Soft S_1
Long PR interval (>200 msec)
Depressed left ventricular contractility
Premature closure of mitral valve (e.g., acute aortic regurgitation)
Left bundle branch block
Extracardiac factors (e.g., obesity, muscular chest, COPD, large breasts)
Flail mitral leaflet

How to Listen to S_1

Timing

Experienced physicians rarely have difficulty identifying S_1 unless there is a rapid heart rate or several murmurs. Tachycardia shortens diastole relatively more than systole. At heart rates of 120–130, systole and diastole are of equal length. If there is any doubt of the proper identification of S_1 and S_2, S_1 should be timed simultaneously with palpation of the carotid pulse or apex impulse.

Characteristics

Typically, S_1 is of medium to high frequency, although occasionally it is low pitched. Use of the diaphragm or increased pressure with the bell will bring out the crisp, high-frequency vibrations of S_1. Splitting of S_1 is audible in many, but not all, normal subjects. S_1 splitting often is better detected medial to the apex or at the lower sternal border. S_1 usually is not prominent at the base and always should be single at the second and third interspaces. *Practical Point: When apparent splitting of S_1 is heard at the base, one should suspect the presence of an ejection sound or early midsystolic click.*

Differentiation of Split S_1 from S_4-S_1 or S_1-Ejection Click

Proper identification of two audible heart sounds close to S_1 provides an important diagnostic challenge to the clinician (Figure 5-1). An S_4 may be confused with the first component of S_1 (see Chapter 6). The S_4 usually is audible only at the apex and often only in the left lateral position. The S_4 is low pitched unless very loud and may be associated with palpable presystolic distention of the left ventricle. An S_4 should attenuate when pressure on the bell of the stethoscope is increased.

An ejection click may be difficult to differentiate from a split S_1 (see Chapter 7). The ejection sound usually is more intense than the second component of S_1 (T_1) and often will be heard well at the base. Splitting of the S_1 is not heard in this area. A pulmonic ejection click usually will vary with respiration. Aortic clicks typically are discrete and snappy at the apex and occur later than the more closely split S_1. The LV apex usually is the site of maximal intensity of the aortic ejection sound.

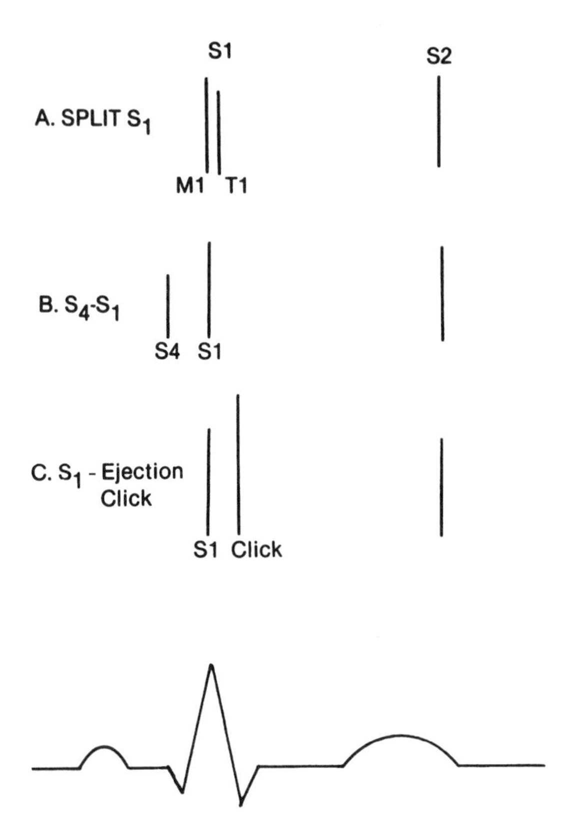

Figure 5-1. Differential diagnosis of audible splitting of the first heart sound: (A) both M_1 and T_1 audible. (B) S_4-S_1 complex. (C) S_1-ejection click complex. Techniques for differentiating these sound combinations are discussed in the text.

Abnormalities of the First Heart Sound

Detectable abnormalities of S_1 on auscultation are few. *Practical Point: The loudness of S_1 provides the most important clinical information in auscultation.* The intensity should be noted and compared to the amplitude of S_2 as well as to other cardiac sounds.

Increased Intensity of S_1

Commonly, S_1 is loud in conditions with increased adrenergic activity or hyperkinetic states such as anemia, exercise, thyrotoxicosis, and anxiety (see Table 5-1). Short PR intervals, such as in the Wolff-Parkinson-White and Lown-Ganong-Levine syndromes, will produce a louder S_1.

Mitral Stenosis
The loud S_1 in rheumatic mitral stenosis is an extremely valuable diagnostic clue (see Chapter 14). S_1 in mitral stenosis usually is palpable at the apex. *Practical Point: A loud S_1 almost always is present in mitral stenosis, except when the mitral valve is so severely fibrosed and calcified that it is virtually immobile. In the absence of a loud S_1, the diagnosis of mitral stenosis should be reconsidered.*

Decreased Intensity of S_1

A soft S_1 is a clue to a long PR interval, which may result in premature mitral valve closure (see Table 5-1). Audible reduction in S_1 amplitude occurs at PR intervals greater than 0.16 sec, and S_1 is markedly attenuated with a PR longer than 0.20 sec. Impaired LV function can produce a decreased S_1. Therefore, S_1 may be soft in patients with congestive heart failure or coronary disease and markedly decreased LV contractility. In aortic valve disease, particularly acute aortic regurgitation, a markedly elevated left ventricular end-diastolic pressure may result in *premature closure* of the mitral valve, reducing the intensity of S_1.

Attenuation in S_1 may result from extracardiac factors such as thick muscular chests, obesity, large breasts, increased thoracic diameter, and chronic obstructive lung disease.

Abnormal Splitting of S_1

Wide splitting of S_1 can result from an electrical delay in ventricular activation, which results in asynchrony of contraction, or from an increase in LV isovolumic contraction time. Right bundle branch block (RBBB), and may produce prominent splitting of S_1; S_2 usually is widely split as well.

Variable S_1

Whenever the relationship between the position of the mitral valve leaflets and LV pressure rise is inconstant, the intensity of S_1 will vary. Therefore, second- or third-degree heart block, AV dissociation, and ventricular rhythms with dissociated atrial rates result in an S_1 of variable intensity.

Second Heart Sound (S_2)

Careful and intelligent evaluation of the intensity and splitting characteristics of the second heart sound (S_2) represents one of the most valuable aspects of cardiac physical diagnosis. Clues to unsuspected or known cardiovascular abnormalities frequently are detected after assessment of S_2. The second heart sound comprises an aortic (A_2) component and a pulmonic (P_2) component; both A_2 and P_2 should be sought separately, identified, and analyzed on auscultation.

Normal Physiology

The two components of S_2 represent vibrations resulting from decleration of the blood mass at the end of ventricular systole when the *semilunar valve cusps coapt* to prevent diastolic reflux of blood (see Figure 1-1). A_2 and P_2 are coincidental with or occur just after the actual closure of the valve cusps.

A_2 and P_2 coincide precisely with the respective incisurae in the aorta and pulmonary artery pressure recordings (see Figure 1-1). The incisura represents the peak deceleration of the blood mass and immediately is followed by a rebound of pressure. The relative distensibility or stiffness of the pulmonary and systemic vascular tree provides a partial explanation for differences in the timing of A_2 and P_2. In the central aorta, resistance is relatively high, compliance is low, and the recoil from the ejection of blood into the aorta is brisk. Consequently, A_2 and its incisura closely follow the end of LV ejection. In the pulmonary artery, the highly distensible, low-resistance pulmonary vasculature allows for a late recoil following right ventricular ejection. Therefore, P_2 and the pulmonary artery incisura are somewhat delayed after the end of RV systole.

Respiratory Effects of A_2 and P_2

Inspiration normally produces audible separation (inspiratory splitting) of A_2 and P_2. The classic view of the mechanism of inspiratory splitting of S_2 is that increased venous return during inspiration causes a delay in RV systole, whereas LV systole remains unchanged or is shortened somewhat; this difference results in an increase in the A_2-P_2 interval. During expiration, RV stroke volume diminishes as LV stroke volume increases; the Q-A_2 interval lengthens and Q-P_2 shortens.

Common Factors Altering S_2

Inspiratory Splitting

Anything that results in either a delay or shortening of right or left ventricular systole or produces an alteration in great vessel impedance and distensibility affects the respiratory relationships of A_2 and P_2. Therefore, disturbances of ventricular electrical activation, abnormal contractile performance, outflow obstruction, or changes in vascular resistance may affect S_2 splitting patterns.

Intensity

The components of S_2 usually have greater acoustic energy and a higher frequency than those of S_1. Elevation of pressure in either great vessel produces a more rapid and forceful deceleration of blood at end systole and results in an S_2 of increased amplitude. Valvular disease often produces the opposite effect: a soft S_2.

How to Listen to S_2

The physician must carefully evaluate the characteristics of *both* A_2 and P_2 during the routine cardiac examination. It is insufficient to assess only the loudness of S_2 at various precordial locations.

Since the major vibrations of S_2 are relatively high pitched, firm or increased pressure on the diaphragm of the stethoscope should be used to auscultate S_2. During expiration, S_2 normally is heard as a single sound. On inspiration, "splitting" or separation of the two components usually can be heard. Most people cannot differentiate two sounds that are only 20–25 msec apart. Therefore, if A_2-P_2 are separated by 20 msec or less, they will be heard as a single sound, such a sound is described as *single* or *fused.*

A_2 is louder than P_2 in normal subjects and in most abnormal states, unless pulmonary hypertension is present or the sound of aortic closure is diminished. A_2 is heard well at the classic aortic area (second right interspace), the pulmonary area (second left interspace), and the cardiac apex. *Practical Point: Normally, only A_2 is audible at the apex, P_2 normally does not radiate to the apex as a separate, audible sound except in young or thin subjects or with pulmonary hypertension.* The normal P_2 is somewhat softer than A_2, even at the pulmonary area, and usually is heard over a relatively small area of the chest. P_2 is readily detected at the second to fourth left interspaces.

S_2 During Respiration

During inspiration, clear-cut separation of A_2 and P_2 normally is observed (Figure 5-2). This splitting is prominent in young subjects but found less predictably in older age groups. P_2 usually becomes maximally delayed in mid- to late inspiration; during expiration, the two components of S_2 are fused or single. Slow regular respirations are best for auscultation. The upright position often accentuates inspiratory separation of A_2 and P_2.

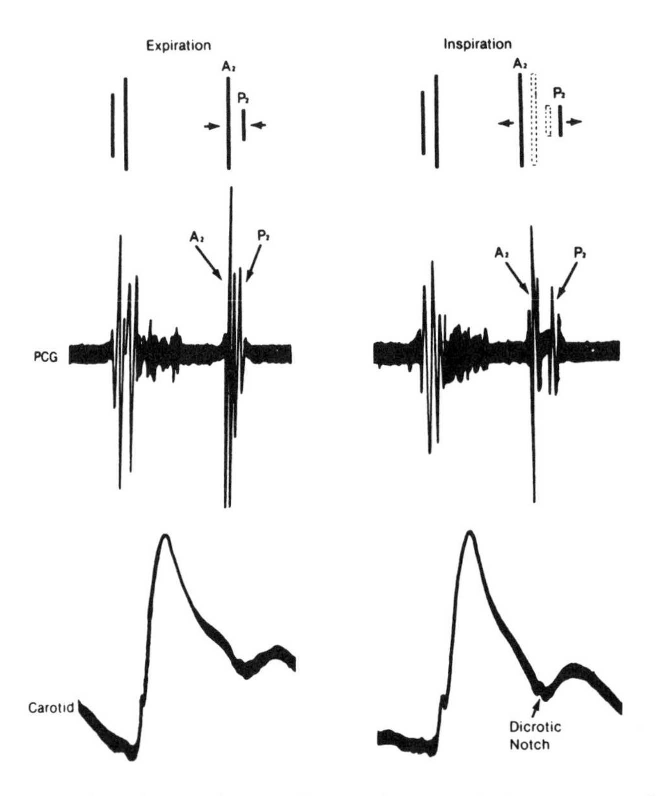

Figure 5-2. Physiologic splitting of S_2. Under normal circumstances, S_2 in expiration is heard as a single event, but in late inspiration, audible splitting of A_2 and P_2 is noted. The normal range of expiratory splitting is from 10–60 msec averaging 40 msec. Most examiners cannot acoustically separate sounds that are 20 msec or less apart; therefore, a narrow splitting interval will be heard as a fused or single S_2. The mechanisms of the inspiratory increase in the A_2-P_2 interval are discussed in the text; the inspiratory increase consists predominantly of an increase in the total Q-P_2 duration.

As the two components separate, a *ta-dup* cadence is heard in inspiration. The average A_2-P_2 splitting interval is 30–40 msec (0.03–0.04 sec), with a range of 10–60 msec. Any interval less than 30 msec is considered "narrow splitting"; in such cases, the two components of S_2 may not be detected and S_2 may seem impure or "dirty" during inspiration.

Detectable expiratory splitting of 40 msec or more usually is abnormal. Any subject who has *audible expiratory splitting* of S_2 in the supine position should be examined sitting or standing (see later). Often S_2 will be muffed in expiration but not discretely split. Asking the subject to hold his or her breath in end expiration may be useful. Younger persons (children and young adults) are more likely to have normal expiratory asynchrony in the supine position and almost always will have prominent inspiratory splitting of S_2. By contrast, normal older subjects rarely have audible expiratory splitting but often have no detectable inspiratory splitting (single S_2).

Body Habitus

In obese subjects, S_2 may be best heard in the first left intercostal space. In tall, thin patients, S_2 may be best appreciated at the lower sternal edge and not the base. In chronic lung disease, the xiphoid area is often the best site for S_2 analysis.

Proper Identification of Systole

During rapid tachycardias or with severe myocardial disease, it may be difficult to distinguish S_1 from S_2. Findings in patients with mitral stenosis or mitral valve prolapse often are confusing. An opening snap and midsystolic click readily can be mistaken for S_1 or S_2, particularly with rapid heart rates (see Figures 14-8 and 15-3). *Practical Point: It is important simultaneously to palpate the carotid artery or the apex impulse when identification of S_1 and S_2 is difficult.*

It is best to begin auscultation at the base; the cadence of S_1 and S_2 is most characteristic at the second to third interspace. Murmurs and other heart sounds usually are sorted out more easily away from the cardiac apex. The inspiratory motion of A_2 and P_2 should identify definitely which sound is S_2. S_1 usually is louder at the apex unless the PR interval is long or LV function is deranged.

Is Splitting of S_2 Present?

In patients with rapid heart rates, particularly infants, the two components of S_2 may be difficult or impossible to hear. In tachypneic patients, the rapid respirations may not allow sufficient time to hear the normal variation in S_2, particularly if the respirations are shallow. During sustained arrhythmias, particularly atrial fibrillation or frequent PVCs, proper evaluation of respiratory splitting can be difficult.

Abnormalities of Second Heart Sound

Intensity

Alterations in the intensity of the loudness of A_2 or P_2 can be valuable in detecting semilunar valvar abnormalities or elevated pressure in one of the great vessels. A particularly loud transient sound often is palpable. For example, a palpable S_2 in the second to third left interspace adjacent to the sternum suggests pulmonary hypertension or, less commonly, systemic hypertension.

Increased A_2

A loud A_2 occurs when there is increased flow or pressure in the central aorta. Aortic root dilatation also can increase the amplitude of A_2. Thickened aortic valve leaflets that retain good mobility may be associated with increased A_2 intensity but more often dampen the amplitude of A_2. In certain congenital lesions involving the great vessels, the aortic closure sound will be increased because the aorta arises more anteriorly than usual or the pulmonary artery is displaced posteriorly (e.g., tetralogy of Fallot).

Increased P_2

The sine qua non of an increased P_2 is pulmonary hypertension. *Practical Point: The observation of an abnormally loud P_2 is one of the most important findings in the cardiac examination and almost always indicates pulmonary hypertension. Since P_2 normally is inaudible at the apex, the occurrence of two audible components of S_2 at the apex strongly suggests pulmonary hypertension and should prompt a careful evaluation of the patient.* In a patient with mitral valve disease or suspected pulmonary vascular or parenchymal disease, a palpable P_2 at the second to third left interspace is a marker for elevated pulmonary pressures. In most patients with pulmonary hypertension, inspiratory splitting is narrower than normal. In an atrial septal defect (ASD) with a large left-to-right shunt, the RV is enlarged; delayed splitting of P_2 often can be heard at the apex in these subjects, even in the absence of elevated PA pressure.

Decreased A_2
In valvar aortic stenosis, aortic closure typically is diminished or absent because of extensive leaflet distortion, fibrosis, or calcification. In aortic regurgitation, A_2 often is diminished.

Decreased P_2
Valvar pulmonic stenosis is associated with a soft or even absent P_2. In addition, P_2 often is delayed in pulmonic stenosis. Augmentation of RV filling by squatting, mild exercise, or leg elevation may increase the intensity of a soft P_2.

Extracardiac Factors
Increased chest wall thickness, significant chest deformity, chronic obstructive lung disease, and obesity can decrease the intensity of all heart sounds. Inspiration often attenuates P_2 by insulation of the pulmonary valve sound due to the interposed lung tissue.

Splitting

Expiratory Splitting
Expiratory splitting refers to the presence of two audible components of S_2 at end expiration. Held expiration may accentuate this finding and induce greater asynchrony. S_2 ordinarily will be heard as a single sound when A_2 and P_2 are separated by 20 msec or less; therefore, audible expiratory splitting indicates an interval of at least 30–40 msec between the two sounds. *Practical Point: RV systole shortens more than LV systole in the sitting or standing position; hence, the respiratory variation of S_2 is enhanced when a subject is upright. In the majority of normal persons who demonstrate expiratory splitting of S_2 in the supine position, S_2 becomes single when the patient sits up.*

Persistence of audible expiratory splitting in the upright position is a valuable clue to an underlying cardiovascular abnormality. Table 5-2 lists conditions that may cause asynchronous right and left ventricular systole and expiratory splitting. Most conditions associated with audible expiratory splitting will demonstrate a further increase in the A_2-P_2 interval with inspiration; if there is no detectable change in the S_2 interval, the split is considered *fixed.*

Delayed P_2 (Increased Q-P_2) Right bundle branch block is the most common cause of expiratory splitting of S_2. S_1 also may be prominently split in RBBB; in this setting, P_2 widens further with inspiration.

Table 5-2. Common Causes of Audible Expiratory Splitting of S_2

Increased Q-P_2
Pulmonic stenosis
Massive pulmonary embolus
Pulmonary hypertension with RV failure
Atrial septal defect
Complete RBBB
PVCs of LV origin
Thoracic skeletal abnormalities
Occasional normals
Decreased Q-A_2
Severe mitral regurgitation
Ventricular septal defect
P_2-A_2 reversal
All causes of paradoxic or reversed splitting (see the text)

Moderate to severe pulmonic stenosis produces delayed splitting of P_2 on expiration; although respiratory motion remains normal, P_2 often is late and may be barely detectable. Audible expiratory splitting often is the first clue to the fixed S_2 of an atrial septal defect. Mild pulmonic stenosis and an ASD are common causes of systolic murmurs in children. The presence of expiratory splitting can be of diagnostic importance in the younger age groups and suggests the presence of an organic cardiac defect.

Decreased Q-A_2 Interval Occasional cases of audible expiratory splitting may be explained by shortened LV systole. This may occur in severe mitral regurgitation, ventricular septal defects, or pericardial tamponade.

Other Causes of Expiratory Splitting Benign causes of expiratory splitting include a minor interventricular conduction delay, pectus excavatum, straight back syndrome, and other musculoskeletal abnormalities. Occasionally, normal children with no evidence of heart disease will display this finding.

Differential Diagnosis of Audible Expiratory Splitting Any complex of sounds consisting of two components in late systole-early diastole may simulate a split S_2 in expiration. Such combinations include an A_2-opening snap, late systolic click-S_2, S_2-pericardial knock, and S_2-S_3 (particularly when the S_3 has high-frequency vibrations).

Wide Inspiratory Splitting

Most of the conditions that produce audible expiratory splitting may also result in a prominent *inspiratory* delay between A_2 and P_2. Occasionally, the respiratory motion of A_2-P_2 is absent when S_2 is widely split; this is known as *fixed splitting.*

Increased Q-P_2 When RV systole is prolonged by either electrical (RBBB, LV pacing) or hemodynamic factors, a prominent delay in P_2 is common. Right ventricular failure from any cause will delay the Q-P_2; in acute and chronic pulmonary embolization, this may be dramatic, even in the absence of RBBB. A similar situation has been described in late pregnancy or advanced renal failure; the delayed Q-P_2 presumably reflects hypervolemia.

In valvular pulmonic stenosis, P_2 is late and the degree of A_2-P_2 delay correlates well with the severity of obstruction. Therefore, an A_2-P_2 interval of 100 msec signifies severe stenosis with an RV-PA gradient greater than 100 mmHg. In atrial septal defects, the large RV stroke volume helps to increase the Q-P_2 interval; an RV conduction defect usually contributes to the delay. The S_2 in patients with an ASD usually is fixed, although respiratory variation occasionally may occur, particularly in the upright position.

In patients with pulmonic stenosis, ASD, or idiopathic dilatation of the pulmonary artery, the Q-P_2 interval is increased.

Decreased Q-A_2 A large ventricular septal defect (VSD) with hyperkinetic pulmonary circulation and normal pulmonary vascular resistance may demonstrate wide inspiratory splitting due to the combination of decreased Q-A_2 and increased Q-P_2 intervals. Patients with constrictive pericarditis, pericardial tamponade, or left atrial myxoma may have wide inspiratory splitting because of shortened LV systole. Shortened LV systole in severe mitral regurgitation is associated with an increased A_2-P_2 interval, particularly if there is associated RV failure.

Fixed Splitting

When right or left ventricular stroke volume does not change during inspiration or when there is a similar degree of respiratory alteration in both RV and LV filling, the splitting of S_2 is fixed. Fixed splitting may occur with a relatively narrow A_2-P_2 interval but is more common (and more noticeable) when the A_2-P_2 interval is wide. Apparent fixed splitting occasionally may be present in young normal patients, but usually disappears when the individual assumes the upright position. *Practical Point: The diagnosis of fixed splitting should be made only after careful auscultation of S_2 in both the recumbent and upright positions.*

Failure to Increase Right Ventricular Stroke Volume with Inspiration Inspiratory augmentation of RV filling may not be possible when there is a major pressure overload of the RV. This is seen in RV failure, acute or chronic pulmonary embolization, and severe pulmonary hypertension (uncommon). In such cases, left ventricular filling also may be subnormal, with a resultant decreased Q-A_2 interval and prominent wide splitting.

Simultaneous Increase in Right Ventricular and Left Ventricular Filling ATRAIL SEPTAL DEFECT. Fixed splitting is the hallmark of ASD. This diagnosis often is first suspected because of the presence of prominent expiratory separation of A_2 and P_2. The right and left atria act as a common venous reservoir; anything that influences RV or LV filling can alter the degree of left-to-right shunting across the atrial defect. The net effect is to "balance out" the respective increases in right and left ventricular filling during inspiration: Both Q-P_2 and Q-A_2 increase simultaneously with no change in the A_2-P_2 splitting interval. Typically, S_2 is widely split. In a small percentage of otherwise typical secundum atrial defects, respiratory splitting is readily detectable. In the pulmonary hypertensive ASD, fixed splitting of S_2 is maintained, although P_2 is markedly increased in intensity.

VENTRICULAR SEPTAL DEFECT. S_2 is normal in the VSD without pulmonary hypertension. In a VSD with markedly elevated pulmonary vascular resistance (Eisenmenger's reaction), the ventricles act as a common chamber. Ejection of blood from both ventricles into the great vessels with an equivalent resistance results in a comparable inspiratory "delay" in each chamber, with absence of respiratory motion of S_2. In most instances, S_2 is fused or single on both inspiration and expiration. This finding is a valuable diagnostic clue, as it strongly suggests that the defect is inoperable.

Differential Diagnosis of Wide Fixed Splitting In patients with LBBB and paradoxic splitting (see later), the presence of congestive heart failure may result in fixed but reversed splitting of S_2 (P_2-A_2). An A_2-opening snap complex in mitral stenosis also can be confused with a widely split S_2, particularly when there is a close A_2-OS interval.

Reversed or Paradoxic Splitting

Reversed splitting occurs when S_2 is maximally split on expiration and narrows or fuses on inspiration (Figure 5-3). Because the directional changes of A_2 and P_2 during the respiratory cycle are reversed from normal, the term *paradoxic splitting* is used widely. In general, this type of splitting is found only when LV electromechanical systole is significantly delayed; that is, an increased Q-A_2 interval. During expiration, prolonged LV systole causes A_2 to follow P_2 (audible expiratory splitting). With inspiration, the Q-P_2 increases normally, but Q-A_2 is unchanged or shortens. The two components of S_2 coincide or occur so close together that the ear appreciates only a single second sound in inspiration.

Causes of Increased Q-A_2 Interval LEFT BUNDLE BRANCH BLOCK. The most common cause of S_2 reversal is left bundle branch block (LBBB). Paradoxic splitting is detectable in most patients with LBBB.

S_2 can be affected by other disorders of LV activation, such as lesser degrees of LBBB (common in left ventricular hypertrophy) and, in some cases, type B Wolff-Parkinson-White syndrome (right ventricular preexcitation from a right-sided bypass tract). Right ventricular pacing and PVCs of right ventricular origin will produce audible paradoxic splitting of S_2.

INCREASED LEFT VENTRICULAR EJECTION TIME. Although relatively uncommon, a large stroke volume in LV volume overload conditions, such as patent ductus arteriosus or severe aortic regurgitation, may result in a prolonged Q-A_2 and reversed splitting. In coronary artery disease or hypertension with acute or chronic LV dysfunction, reversed splitting of S_2 occasionally is noted, although it is uncommon.

LEFT VENTRICULAR OUTFLOW TRACT OBSTRUCTION. Reversed splitting may be observed in valvular aortic stenosis and hypertrophic cardiomyopathy. Splitting of S_2 in hypertrophic cardiomyopathy may vary from normal to paradoxic in the same patient from day to day.

Clue to Auscultation of Reversed Splitting The physician should listen carefully over *many* respiratory cycles to be certain S_2 moves paradoxically. When the respiratory splitting pattern remains unclear, Constant suggests careful assessment of the amplitude of both components of S_2 as the stethoscope is moved from base to apex. The component that softens as the stethoscope approaches the apex will be P_2; this should clarify whether the S_2 sequence is A_2-P_2 or P_2-A_2.

Pseudoparadoxic Splitting Deep inspiration, particularly in subjects with large chests or chronic obstructive lung disease, may cause an

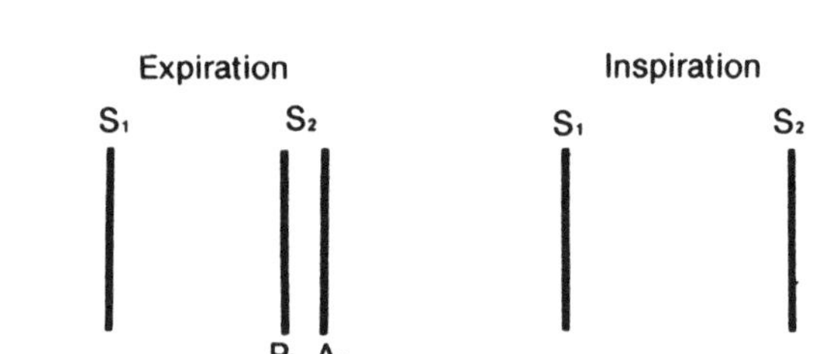

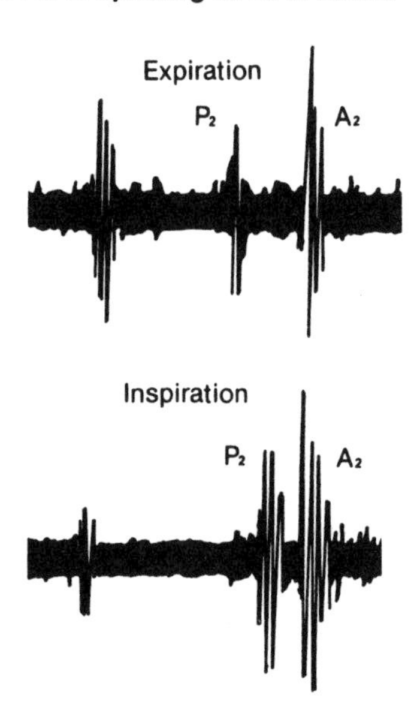

Figure 5-3. Reversed or paradoxic splitting of the second heart sound. The usual cause of paradoxic splitting is abnormally delayed left ventricular ejection, such that aortic closure (A_2) follows pulmonic closure (P_2). This commonly results in audible expiratory splitting. During inspiration, the normal delay in the Q-P_2 interval results in P_2 "moving into" A_2, and a single or narrower S_2 occurs. Thus, the normal respiratory pattern is reversed.

artifactual muffling or disappearance of P_2 due to interposition of the expanded lung between the stethoscope and the aorta. If S_2 is audibly split in expiration, this phenomenon may result in the false diagnosis of reversed or paradoxic splitting, as S_2 appears to become "single" in inspiration.

Single (or Narrow) Splitting of S_2
A single S_2 will be heard on inspiration when either A_2 or P_2 is inaudible or when the inspiratory separation of A_2 and P_2 is so narrow (less than 30 msec) that the ear cannot distinguish both components. The patient should be examined in both reclining and sitting positions to confirm the presence of a single S_2. Care must be taken to avoid irregular, rapid, and shallow respirations; ask the patient to breathe slowly and deeply. The following are common causes of a single S_2.

Aging The incidence of audible inspiratory splitting of S_2 in normal subjects decreases with age. In up to 50% of subjects over 60 years of age, S_2 is single.

Artifactual Muffling of P_2 This results from lung insulation of P_2 during inspiration and is more common in older people.

Reversed Splitting In conditions associated with reversed splitting, an equal duration of systole in both ventricles may cause S_2 to be heard as single in both phases of respiration. Reversed or paradoxic splitting of S_2 should be readily distinguishable from a single S_2 by detection of expiratory separation of A_2 and P_2 in expiration.

Pulmonary Hypertension In subjects with marked elevation of PA pressure and good RV function, a narrow A_2-P_2 interval is the rule, and S_2 may appear to be single in inspiration (see Figure 7-4).

Masking P_2 can be masked in the presence of a high-intensity, closely split sound of aortic closure or a loud mitral opening snap.

Murmur Obscuration Long or holosystolic murmurs such as those of mitral regurgitation, ventricular septal defect, aortic stenosis, pulmonic stenosis, or patent ductus arteriosus can engulf or mask either A_2 or P_2. In these situations, careful listening at the apex and lower left sternal border for A_2 and P_2 is necessary. It often is useful to listen to the behavior of the S_2 splitting away from the site of maximal murmur intensity.

6

The Third and Fourth Heart Sounds

The presence of a third (S_3) or fourth (S_4) heart sound may be extremely important in the evaluation of adults with suspected or known cardiovascular disease. An S_3 may be a normal or abnormal finding; the presence of an S_3 in an adult over 40 may have serious implications about the status of left ventricular function, but in a young subject this finding usually is normal. An audible S_4 generally is present only in abnormal hearts.

Third Heart Sound

Physiology of S_3

The S_3 follows mitral valve opening and the onset of rapid ventricular filling (Figure 6-1). Rapid deceleration of blood during inflow to the left ventricle is translated into vibratory energy, resulting in the S_3. The relaxing ventricle and increasing diastolic blood volume set the ventricular walls, mitral valve apparatus, and blood mass into vibration.

The intensity of S_3 is increased when early diastolic filling is rapid due to elevated left atrial pressure or blood volume or when left ventricular distensibility in early diastole is increased. When LV compliance

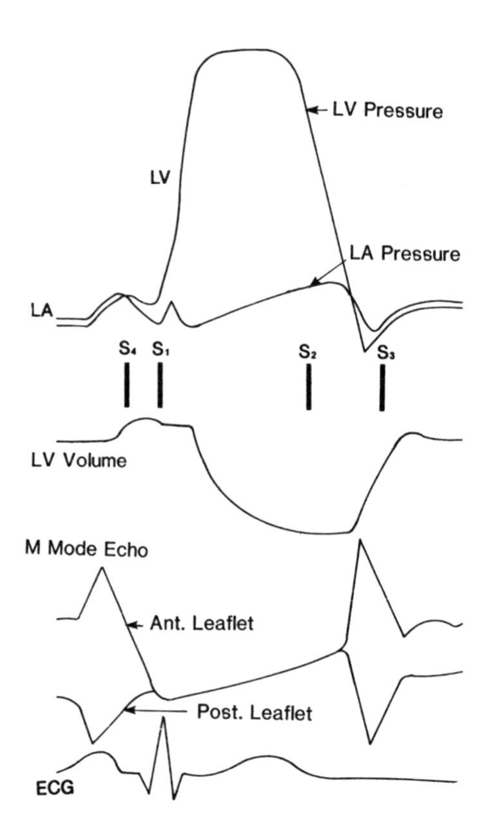

Figure 6-1. Intracardiac pressure, mitral valve motion, and left ventricular volume interrelationships in heart sound generation. Left ventricular and left atrial pressures are displayed with the simultaneous M-mode echo and left ventricular volume in relation to the four heart sounds. Note the timing of the heart sounds with respect to left atrial-left ventricular pressure crossover, mitral leaflet motion, and alterations in left ventricular volume.

is decreased, the rate of early diastolic filling is decreased; in these situations, S_3 may not be present but an S_4 may be audible (see page 84).

The physiologic explanation for the presence of an S_3 in normal children and young adults but not in older subjects is unclear. An S_3 also may be produced in the right ventricle when there is RV dysfunction or excessive flow across the tricuspid valve. Whether the right ventricle contributes to the normal or physiologic S_3 is unknown.

The S_3 sometimes is called a *ventricular gallop, early diastolic gallop* or *sound,* or *S_3 gallop*. Although the term *S_3* or *third heart sound* is preferred, *ventricular gallop* is acceptable when there is definite underlying heart disease.

Clinical Significance of the Third Heart Sound

An S_3 may be present in (1) normal hearts, (2) diastolic overload states, and (3) patients who have LV dysfunction, with or without overt congestive heart failure (Table 6-1).

Normal Hearts

An S_3 commonly is found in normal children and young adults. Although not usually present in healthy subjects over 40 years of age, an S_3 occasionally may be found in individuals in their 30s (especially in women) without evidence of cardiac disease. In states such as

Table 6-1. Clinical Correlates of the Third Heart Sound

Normal or physiologic S_3
Children, young adults
Hyperkinetic states in subjects with normal hearts
Diastolic overload states
Left ventricle
Mitral regurgitation
Ventricular septal defect
Patent ductus arteriosus
Right ventricle
Tricuspid regurgitation
Atrial septal defect (uncommon)
Left ventricle dysfunction
Congestive heart failure
Dilated left ventricle
Markedly depressed ejection fraction
Constrictive pericarditis
Pericardial knock

anemia, thyrotoxicosis, anxiety, exercise, and pregnancy, a physiologic S_3 may become more prominent or appear for the first time.

Normal Heart with Increased Cardiac Output
In the normal heart with increased cardiac output and augmented velocity of diastolic filling, an audible "physiologic" S_3 may be present, which is acoustically indistinguishable from a pathologic ventricular gallop. The S_3 may be soft or loud and usually attenuates or disappears when the subject assumes the upright position. Most individuals with a physiologic S_3 are young and may have associated systolic flow murmurs or a venous hum. *Practical Point: In children and young adults, it is important to consider the possibility that an S_3 is physiologic and related to increased cardiac output. This will avoid the false diagnosis of cardiac disease.* Occasionally, a physiologic S_3 will be sustained in duration and can simulate a short diastolic murmur. In the thin subject or a child with a hyperactive heart, a normal S_3 actually may be palpable.

Diastolic Overload States

An S_3 may be produced whenever an increased volume of left atrial blood crosses the mitral valve in early diastole, especially if left atrial pressure is increased. Therefore, an S_3 is likely to be found in hemodynamically significant mitral regurgitation, ventricular septal defects, or a patent ductus arteriosus. In mitral regurgitation, the S_3 characteristically is somewhat earlier than usual and may have dominant high frequency vibrations simulating an opening snap.

The S_3 in diastolic overload states is acoustically similar to the normal S_3. Left-to-right shunts with increased mitral valve flow (e.g., patent ductus arteriosus, ventricular septal defect) and mitral regurgitation commonly produce loud diastolic filling sounds (S_3), often with short aftervibrations or a mid-diastolic flow rumble. These can be soft or prominent. If LV contractile function is normal, the S_3 has no ominous prognosis but does indicate a major volume overload.

Tricuspid regurgitation does not produce a prominent S_3 unless there is an enormous RV volume overload. Atrial septal defects usually are not associated with a loud S_3, although a mid-diastolic flow rumble is common in patients with a large left-to-right shunt.

Left Ventricular Dysfunction

An S_3 is characteristic of global LV impairment. In a middle-aged or older adult without mitral regurgitation, the presence of an S_3

suggests a significant decrease in myocardial contractility and a depressed ejection fraction. If the S_3 is related to a new clinical event (e.g., accelerated hypertension, acute myocardial infarction), the S_3 may be transient and disappear when LV function improves.

Significant myocardial disease of any etiology may result in an abnormal S_3. In the presence of left ventricular decompensation associated with functional mitral regurgitation, the S_3 may be related more to the poor ventricular function than to the left atrial volume overload. In such cases, the systolic murmur tends to be soft and the heart larger than in patients with primary mitral regurgitation and good left ventricular function.

A pathologic S_3 caused by LV decompensation will persist when the patient assumes the upright position, although it may soften with this maneuver. The S_3 may be very loud and often is associated with other signs of LV decompensation, such as pulsus alternans, a sustained LV apical impulse, narrow pulse pressure, or signs of overt congestive heart failure. In general, a persistent and loud S_3 heralds a poor prognosis.

An S_3 in the presence of coronary artery disease strongly suggests major LV asynergy or an LV aneurysm. A sustained LV lift or ectopic impulse is a common associated finding. An S_3 gallop is common in decompensated hypertensive and aortic valve disease. A loud S_3 is typical of dilated cardiomyopathy but is not found in hypertrophic cardiomyopathy.

Pericardial Knock of Constrictive Pericarditis

The early, loud, and high-pitched diastolic sound often associated with constrictive pericarditis actually is an "S_3" that occurs earlier than the typical S_3 (0.08–0.10 sec after A_2). The pericardial knock usually has a clicking or snappy quality and easily is mistaken for an opening snap. The early and prominent pericardial knock or S_3 is related to an elevated left atrial pressure and a rapid rise of early ventricular diastolic pressure caused by the nondistensible pericardial shell encasing the heart or the extremely stiff myocardium of restrictive cardiomyopathy.

Fourth Heart Sound

Although there is no disagreement about the mechanism of production of the S_4, considerable controversy concerns its true incidence and clinical implications.

Physiology of S_4

The S_4 is a low frequency sound following left atrial systole (see Figure 6-1). Although also known as the *atrial sound*, the S_4 is ventricular in origin. Audible vibrations of the S_4 result from sudden tensing of the LV mass, the mitral valve apparatus, and the blood within the ventricle. It follows the P wave by 0.14–0.20 sec and precedes S_1.

The *hemodynamic correlates* of the abnormal S_4 include an LV chamber that often is hypertrophied but with little or no increase in LV diameter, normal LV pressure in early diastole with an elevation of *end-diastolic pressure*, impaired velocity of early LV diastolic filling, and well-preserved cardiac output. The LV chamber is stiff and noncompliant.

Normal S_4

An S_4 occasionally may be heard despite no detectable abnormalities of ventricular function other than increased blood flow, as in young subjects or patients with thyrotoxicosis or in the presumed physiologic loss of left ventricular compliance with aging. Whether a distinct audible S_4 truly is normal in older adults remains the subject of controversy.

Abnormal S_4

In the normal heart, the LV passively receives 70–80% of its diastolic filling volume from the left atrium during early to middiastole, with a smaller contribution from atrial contraction in late diastole. In myocardial disease such as hypertrophy or dilatation, left atrial contraction becomes responsible for a greater proportion of LV filling. This LA "booster pump" function takes on increasing importance as LV distensibility decreases: Left atrial contraction may provide up to 30–40% of LV diastolic filling in some circumstances. Under these conditions, the S_4 or atrial gallop may be prominent (analogous to P wave enlargement on the EKG). Early to mid-LV diastolic pressure usually is normal, but LV end-diastolic pressure is elevated. The S_4 often is palpable in these circumstances.

Importance of Left Atrial Function

Vigorous left atrial contraction is necessary to provide sufficient blood flow to abruptly distend the LV in late diastole and produce an audible S_4. In chronic severe mitral regurgitation, an S_4 is rare in spite of elevated left atrial pressure; the left atrium is large and distensible, atrial contractile force is diminished. When the onset of mitral regurgitation is acute or recent, however, an S_4 is common: The normal-sized atrium contracts with a greatly increased force (see Chapter 13, Figure 13-6).

Prevalence of S_4: An Unresolved Controversy

In recent years, two major unresolved issues regarding the S_4 have been the subject of considerable debate. These relate to the *audibility* of the S_4 and the *normality* of finding an atrial sound in adults. These questions are relevant because of numerous observations that phonocardiograms record an S_4 at the cardiac apex in many adults with no evidence of overt heart disease. General consensus accepts that a *very loud* or *palpable S_4* always is abnormal and signifies decreased LV compliance (Figure 6-2). *Practical Point: The majority of clinicians and investigators believe that the presence of a distinctly audible atrial sound or S_4 in an older subject almost always is abnormal and, conversely, that normal persons infrequently have a distinctly audible S_4.*

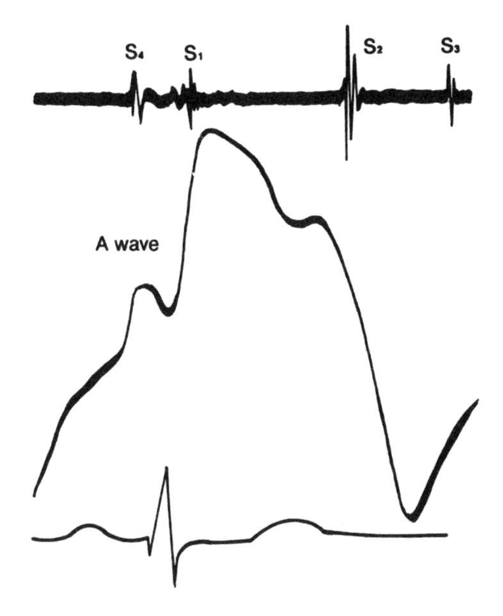

Figure 6-2. Palpable atrial sound. Careful examination of the left ventricular apex beat may reveal that a very loud S_4 is associated with a palpable presystolic impulse. This is more likely to be found when patients are turned into the left lateral decubitus position. The presence of a palpable S_4 indicates that the atrial sound is pathologic.

Clinical Significance

A prominent S_4, often with a palpably increased precordial A wave amplitude, commonly is found in patients with underlying coronary disease, hypertension, aortic stenosis, or hypertrophic cardiomyopathy. The intensity of an S_4 varies considerably: When prominent, the S_4 may be the loudest heart sound heard at the apex. The common denominator in individuals with a prominent S_4 is left ventricular hypertrophy with increased LV end-diastolic pressure and restricted early diastolic filling produced by a stiff left ventricle. The clinical implication of an audible S_4 is far different from that of the S_3, which often signifies cardiac decompensation, incipient or overt congestive heart failure, and a poor long-term outlook. In general, an S_4 implies a less serious alteration in left ventricular function and carries a more benign prognosis than the S_3.

Clinical Correlates

Normal Hearts

An atrial sound occasionally may be heard in normal children and young adults. Hyperkinetic states, such as anemia or thyrotoxicosis, are likely to produce an audible S_4.

PR Interval

Subjects with a long PR interval (first degree AV block) may have an audible S_4 in the absence of other evidence of cardiovascular disease. S_1 is loud with short PR intervals (see Chapter 5).

Coronary Heart Disease

An S_4 is a hallmark of ischemic heart disease. For instance, the reduced LV compliance resulting from a previous myocardial infarction frequently results in an audible S_4. An audible S_4 has been demonstrated in 80–90% of patients during acute myocardial infarction. The S_4 initially may be inaudible in the acute infarct patient but usually will be manifest after one or two days. Experienced clinicians commonly hear atrial gallops in patients with angina or prior myocardial infarction. In patients with LV asynergy or an overt LV aneurysm, an S_4 is common and typically palpable.

Hypertension

An isolated S_4 is common in chronic hypertension, suggesting LV hypertrophy and reduced compliance even in the absence of definite EKG evidence of LVH. In this setting, the S_4 does not indicate serious left ventricular dysfunction.

Aortic Stenosis

An audible S_4 in patients with valvar aortic stenosis may be a valuable sign, indicating a significant left ventricular aortic gradient. The finding of an S_4 in patients over 50, however, is less specific in predicting severe aortic stenosis, as coronary disease or hypertension frequently may cause an S_4 in this age group. A palpable or extremely loud atrial sound in aortic stenosis usually indicates severe aortic valve obstruction in any group (see Figure 10-4).

Hypertrophic Cardiomyopathy

Audible and palpable atrial sounds almost always are present in hypertrophic cardiomyopathy; if an S_4 is absent, the diagnosis should be seriously questioned. Often a huge precordial A wave is the dominant outward impulse. An S_4 is characteristic of both obstructive and nonobstructive varieties of hypertrophic cardiomyopathy.

Cardiomyopathy

An S_4 may be heard or palpable in subjects with significant myocardial disease. An S_3 also typically is present and in late stages is more likely to be present than an S_4.

Acute Mitral Regurgitation

An S_4 is characteristic of patients with mitral regurgitation of recent onset. The acute left atrial volume overload results in a forceful atrial contraction that expels blood into a normal-sized left ventricle and a resultant atrial sound. The presence of an S_4 in a patient with mitral regurgitation strongly suggests that the mitral lesion is relatively new.

Right Ventricular S_4

In pulmonary hypertension and pulmonary stenosis, a right-sided S_4 is common. The presence of an S_4 in a patient suspected of pulmonary embolization is an important finding, suggesting a significant RV pressure overload. Inspiratory augmentation of the S_4 and maximal location at the lower left sternal border are helpful in the differential diagnosis of a right ventricular S_4.

Summation Gallop and Quadruple Rhythm

Whenever the PR interval is long or the heart rate rapid, atrial contraction will "move into" the rapid filling phase of diastole. Since the diastole shortens more than the systole when the heart rate increases, passive ventricular filling is superimposed on the augmented flow across the mitral valve due to the LA systole. This combination may cause a very loud *summation* gallop (S_3 plus S_4). Cardiac slowing with carotid sinus massage is a useful bedside technique to evaluate gallop rhythm during tachycardia or to help analyze other confusing cardiac findings during a rapid heart rate.

When both an S_3 and S_4 are clearly audible, the term *quadruple rhythm* is used. This commonly is found in patients with LV aneurysm, cardiomyopathy, severe LV failure, or LV dilatation.

How to Listen for S_3 and S_4

The third and fourth heart sounds are low pitched (20–60 cps) and usually of low intensity. They occur at the lower range of human audibility at a frequency range below which most people are accustomed to hearing cardiac sound. The S_3 often has some "duration" or aftervibrations; the S_4 is slightly higher pitched and usually is louder.

Both sounds must be actively sought in order to be detected. They typically sound like a distant thud. The sounds may be palpable, particularly the S_4. To hear the S_3 and S_4 best, a noise-free room with no background vibrations from air conditioning or heating systems is desirable (Table 6-2). Avoid sound artifacts from muscle tremor or interfering noises from clothing or stethoscope tubing.

The S_3 and S_4 often are best heard immediately upon beginning auscultation and may appear to fade away after a short period. Frequently, gallop sounds are heard only immediately after the patient assumes a new position, such as getting onto the examining table or turning over into the left lateral position.

Timing and Respiratory Variation

The S_3 is linked to S_2 in timing, whereas the S_4 occurs just before S_1 (see Figure 6-1); these relationships hold for very slow or very rapid

Table 6-2. Proper Approach to Auscultation of S_3 and S_4

Means	Response
Stethoscope technique	
Room and surroundings quiet	
Routinely use left lateral position	
Identify LV apex impulse	
Use the bell with light pressure	
Use rubber outer ring on bell	
Helpful physiologic maneuvers	
Alterations in venous return	
Increase leg elevation, coughing, situps, abdominal compression, Valsalva release phase	Increase intensity
Decrease: sitting, standing, Valsalva strain phase	Decrease intensity
Sustained handgrip (isometric)	Increase intensity
If heart rate is rapid, use carotid sinus massage	

heart rates. The S_3 occurs in early diastole, usually 0.14–0.16 sec after A_2 (the range is 0.10–0.20 sec). The S_4 is presystolic: It follows the P wave by 0.12–0.20 sec, and immediately precedes S_1 (see Figure 6-1). The S_3 may vary with respiration and usually is loudest during expiration, fading at end inspiration.

Helpful Maneuvers in Auscultation of S_3 and S_4

Maneuvers that alter venous return are useful during auscultation of the low-frequency diastolic filling sounds (see Table 6-2). Anything that increases venous return and intracardiac blood volume accentuates the loudness of S_3 and S_4; conversely, a decrease in cardiac filling will attenuate these sounds. A right-sided S_3 or S_4 will augment with inspiration. Having the patient assume an upright posture often is helpful; both an S_3 and an S_4 typically attenuate or disappear. Carotid sinus pressure may be effective in slowing the heart rate when there is difficulty in timing the gallop rhythm. Handgrip exercise may increase the intensity of both the S_3 and S_4.

Proper Use of the Stethoscope

The S_3 and S_4 are low-frequency transients best and often heard only with the bell of the stethoscope. A large diameter bell with a rubber outer ring is best (see Figure 1-1). The lightest possible pressure to make a skin seal should be used. As stethoscope pressure is increased to filter out low frequency vibrations, the S_3 and S_4 will attenuate. A particularly loud S_3 or S_4 usually has medium- to high-frequency components that may sound higher pitched than usual and remain audible even when firm stethoscope pressure is applied.

Location

The LV S_3 and S_4 are maximal at the apex impulse. The apical impulse should be carefully identified with the examining finger (see Figure 4-4), then the bell should be placed directly on the apex using light pressure (Figure 6-3). In patients with emphysema, the LV S_3 or S_4 may be heard best at the subxiphoid area or lower left sternal border. Differentiation from gallops of RV origin in these patients may be difficult.

Left Lateral Decubitus Position

It is essential to examine any patient suspected of having left ventricular disease in the left oblique or left lateral decubitus position (see Figures 4-4 and 6-3). *Practical Point: The S_3 and S_4 often are inaudible when the patient is supine and may be heard only in the left lateral position.* This maneuver thrusts the apex of the left ventricle close to the chest wall and accentuates audibility of low-pitched diastolic sounds, often increasing dramatically the amplitude of both the S_3 and S_4. In this position, these low-frequency events may become palpable; light pressure on the pads of the fingers should be used, with careful attention for a presystolic bulge or an early systolic thrust. A palpable presystolic distention (S_4) is much more common than a palpable S_3 and a most important confirmatory finding in patients with a suspected S_4 (see Figure 6-2).

Right Ventricular Origin of S_3 and S_4

Any condition resulting in right ventricular hypertrophy or dilatation may produce a right-sided diastolic heart sound. The cardinal features of an S_3 and S_4 generated in the right heart are (1) maximal intensity at the lower left sternal border (tricuspid area), (2) inspiratory augmentation, and (3) evidence for associated right ventricular disease (e.g., parasternal lift, increased P_2, elevated jugular venous pressure

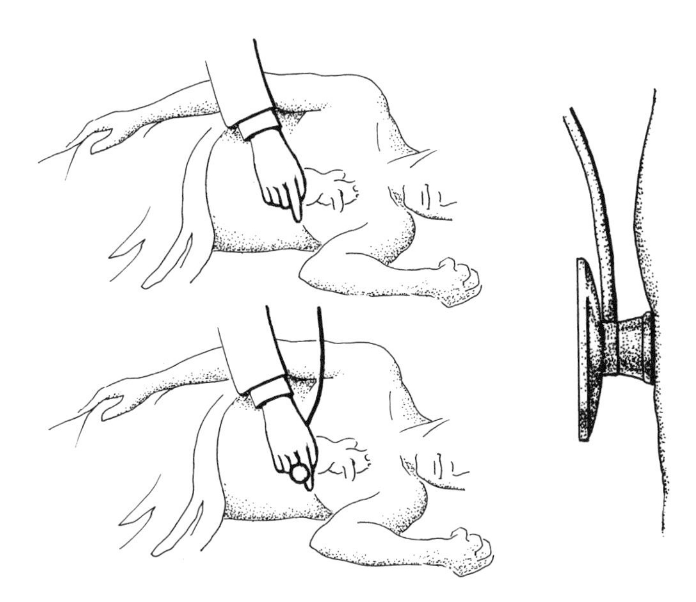

Figure 6-3. Use of the left lateral decubitus position in detection of S_3 and S_4: (top) the left ventricular apex first is identified by careful palpation; (bottom) the bell of the stethoscope then is applied directly over the apical impulse, using the lightest pressure possible that will create a skin seal. This technique enhances audibility of low-frequency cardiac sounds, such as S_3, S_4, mitral diastolic murmurs.

with large A or V waves). A right-sided S_4 is common in the presence of pulmonary hypertension, which results in right ventricular hypertrophy with decreased compliance.

Auscultation of S_4

Many important aspects of proper auscultation of the S_4 have been discussed. Several points require emphasis:

1. The S_4 frequently is audible *only* in the left lateral position and must be sought carefully in any patient with suspected LV disease.
2. Confusion between a split S_1 or S_1-ejection click complex is common. Most double sounds heard at the apex in the adult represent a split S_1 and not an S_4-S_1 complex.

3. The S_4 often is palpable in the left decubitus position; this finding indisputably confirms that the S_4 is an abnormal event in a given patient.
4. Other signs of cardiovascular disease (e.g., increased venous A wave, LV heave) may influence the examiner's impression regarding the presence or absence of S_4. Complete objectivity is important as one assesses all clues that suggest underlying cardiovascular disease.

Differential Diagnosis of S_4

When two sounds in close proximity are heard at the apex at the time of S_1, the differential diagnosis includes a prominently split S_1, an S_4-S_1 complex, and an S_1-early click complex (see Table 7-1).

S_4-S_1 Complex

The S_4 is the first of the two sounds; it is low pitched and may vary with respiration. The S_4, but not the S_1, will attenuate or disappear with firm pressure on the stethoscope bell; it becomes softer in the upright position. The S_4 may be heard only in the left lateral position. It usually is a duller sound than S_1, but when the S_4 is loud, it may become medium-high pitched. An S_4 often is palpable.

Split S_1

Splitting of S_1 is audible at the apex, but the two components of S_1 usually are more discrete at the lower left sternal border. Only a single S_1 is heard at the base. The two components of S_1 are best heard with the diaphragm. The intensity of a split S_1 does not vary when the subject sits or stands, whereas an S_4 softens with the upright position.

S_1-Ejection Click

An S_1-ejection click complex is more easily confused with a split S_1 than the S_4-S_1 combination, and these two sounds infrequently simulate an S_4-S_1 complex (see Table 7-1). Both S_1 and ejection clicks are medium- to high-pitched sounds. A pulmonic ejection sound will vary prominently with respiration. Aortic ejection clicks usually are best heard at the apex; the pulmonic click is loudest at the upper sternal edge and is not audible at the apex.

Palpable S_4

Careful palpation of the apical impulse in the left decubitus position may be rewarded by detection of an outward presystolic thrust in patients with a palpable S_4 (see Chapter 4 and Figures 4-4 and 6-2). This motion often is subtle; commonly, it feels as if there is a shelf or notch on the upstroke of the apex impulse.

The palpable A wave occurs just before the maximal outward apical excursion during isovolumic systole. Two fingers should be used for detection of a palpable S_4. It is important to feel the apex beat over many cardiac cycles, as the size of maximum impulse may alter slightly with respiration and the low amplitude A wave may not be palpable with each heart beat. *Practical Point: The finding of a palpable S_4 indicates that the associated atrial sound definitely is abnormal.*

7

Ejection Sounds

Ejection sounds are high-frequency transients that occur in early systole immediately following the first heart sound (S_1) (Figure 7-1). They also are known as *ejection clicks*; either term is acceptable. Ejection sounds (ES) occur more frequently than commonly is realized. Unless the observer is aware of the possibility of such acoustic events, the ES easily can be assumed to be a part of S_1 and completely missed. The finding of an ejection click may be the critical clue that a systolic murmur is truly organic and almost always implies underlying cardiovascular disease.

Pathophysiology of Ejection Sounds

Two different mechanisms may result in an ejection click: (1) the snapping open or doming of a stenotic thickened or malformed *pulmonary* or *aortic valve* (Figure 7-2A) or (2) a sound transient produced by sudden tensing or reverberation of the proximal *aorta* or *pulmonary artery* at the time of early ejection (vascular or root origin; Figure 7-2B). Ejection clicks of valve origin classically are found in congenital aortic and pulmonary artery valve stenosis. Aortic and pulmonary ejection sounds of the nonstenotic valve variety invariably are associated with either a dilated aorta or pulmonary artery or a systemic or pulmonary vascular tree with an increased systolic pressure and reduced vascular compliance.

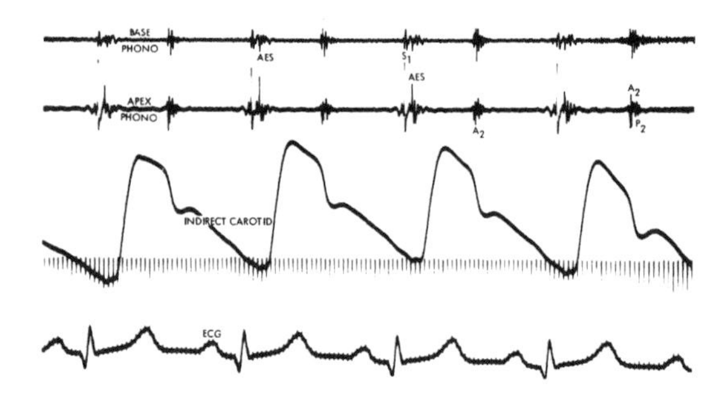

Figure 7-1. Aortic ejection sound. This phonocardiogram and carotid arterial pulse tracing demonstrates a prominent, discrete aortic ejection sound that is heard and recorded better at the apex than at the base. This is characteristic of aortic ejection sounds or clicks. Note the prominent separation of the ejection sound from S_1 by approximately 40–50 msec. (Reprinted with permission from Shaver JA, Griff FW, and Leonard JJ. Ejection sounds of left-sided origin. In: Leon DF, Shaver JA, eds. *Physiologic Principles of Heart Sounds and Murmurs*. American Heart Association Monograph No. 46. Armonk, NY: Futura; 1975.)

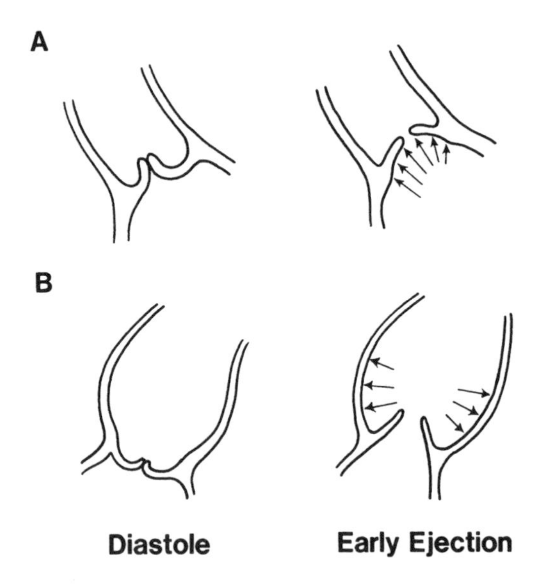

Figure 7-2. Origin of ejection sounds: (A) Ejection sound or click produced by the opening motion of a thickened, often stenotic aortic or pulmonary valve; (B) ejection sound produced by sudden tensing of the proximal aorta or pulmonary artery during early ejection, usually associated with a dilated or hypertensive great vessel (see text).

Semilunar Valve Stenosis

When commissural fusion of a semilunar valve or leaflet thickening is present, the rapidly rising ventricular pressure in early systole drives the abnormal valve leaflets upward. At the precise moment of maximum ascent, the taut valve cusps bulge or dome into their respective great vessel, producing a high-frequency sound (see Figure 7-2A). Flow across the stenotic valve occurs only after maximal valve opening has been reached, and the resultant systolic ejection murmur immediately follows the ejection click. When the valve stenosis is extremely severe and the valve cusps are relatively immobile, both the ES and the respective valve component of S_2 are diminished or even absent. Extensive calcification, as frequently found in aortic stenosis, is another major cause of inaudibility of both an ejection click and its S_2 counterpart.

Aortic Stenosis

An ejection click is almost always present in congenital abnormalities of the aortic valve (see Figure 10-3). Most often, an aortic ES indicates a bicuspid aortic valve. Often, an isolated ejection click may be heard in the absence of an ejection murmur (see Figure 7-1); echocardiography is mandatory in these situations to assess the possibility of a bicuspid or otherwise thickened aortic valve. In *acquired* aortic valve stenosis, usually of rheumatic or degenerative origin, ejection clicks are much less common.

Pulmonic Stenosis

Ejection sounds are common in valvular pulmonic stenosis. As with the aortic valve, the presence of an ES localizes the obstruction to valve level. Infundibular pulmonic stenosis does not produce an ejection click. In very mild or very severe pulmonic stenosis, the pulmonic ejection click may not be heard. *Practical Point: The most characteristic attribute of the pulmonic valve ejection sound is its marked variability with respiration.* In contradistinction to almost all other right-sided acoustic phenomena, which become louder with inspiration, the pulmonic valve ejection click typically *softens* or *disappears* with inspiration (Figure 7-3).

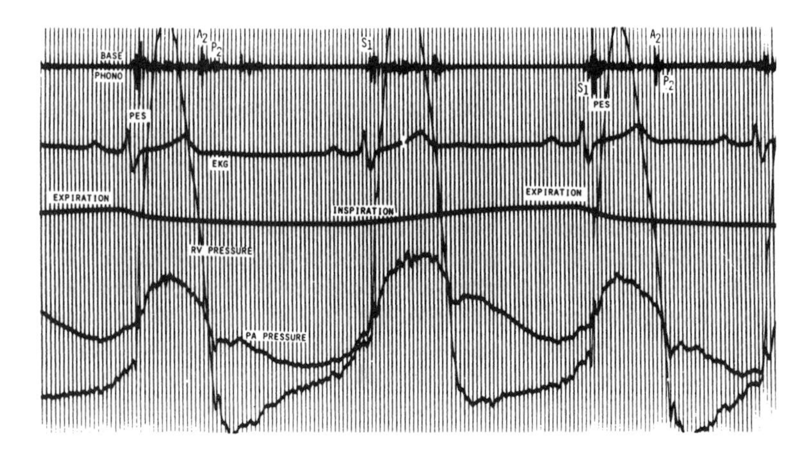

Figure 7-3. Mechanism of the pulmonic ejection sound in pulmonic stenosis. During inspiration right ventricular (RV) end-diastolic pressure exceeds pulmonary artery diastolic pressure, producing an upward opening movement of the pulmonic valve cusps prior to actual ejection. Therefore, the valve already assumes a partially "domed" position and undergoes less upward excursion during early systole; the ejection sound attenuates or completely disappears. (Reprinted with permission from Shaver JA, Griff FW, and Leonard JJ. Ejection sounds of left-sided origin. In: Leon DF, Shaver JA, eds. *Physiologic Principles of Heart Sounds and Murmurs.* American Heart Association Monograph No. 46. Armonk, NY: Futura; 1975.)

Nonvalvular Ejection Sounds

An ES with a normal semilunar valve typically is associated with dilatation of the aorta or pulmonary artery, which occurs in conditions of an increased stroke volume or force of ejection (see Figure 7-2B).

Aortic Root Ejection Sounds

These sounds are found in subjects with aortic arteriosclerosis, aortic aneurysm, aortic regurgitation, or systemic hypertension.

Pulmonary Ejection Sounds

Pulmonary ejection sounds may occur in any condition resulting in pulmonary hypertension (Figure 7-4). In such situations, the respiratory variation of the pulmonic ES is not common. Early ejection of blood into a tense, noncompliant pulmonary artery is thought to be the cause of the ES.

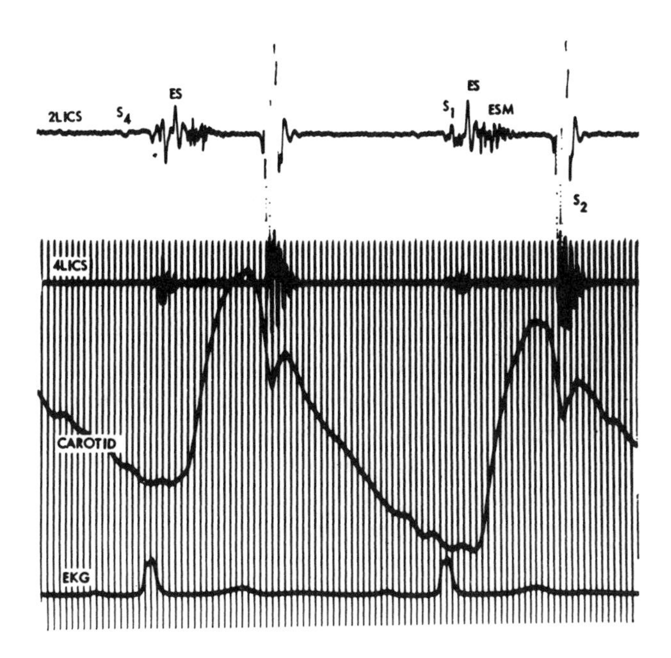

Figure 7-4. Pulmonary ejection sound (ES) in pulmonary hypertension. This phonocardiogram was taken from a patient with pulmonary hypertension due to an Eisenmenger ventricular septal defect. S_2 is single and accentuated. In this situation, the pulmonic ejection click is believed to originate from the dilated and tense pulmonary artery and not from the pulmonary valve itself. ESM = early systolic murmur (see Figure 7-2B). (Reprinted with permission from Reddy PS, Shaver JA, Leonard JJ. Cardiac systolic murmurs; pathophysiology and differential diagnosis. *Prog Cardiovasc Dis.* 1971;14:1.)

Clues to Auscultation of Ejection Sounds

Quality and Timing

Both aortic and pulmonic ejection clicks typically are high-frequency, sharp, discrete sounds at least equal in intensity to S_1 (see Figures 7-1, 7-3, 7-4, and 10-3). They are heard best with the diaphragm of the stethoscope. The later the ejection sound, the more audible it is. Ejection sounds distinctly separate acoustically from S_1 follow the first heart sound by at least 0.05 sec. The opening clicks of stenotic semilunar valves occur later in systole than those of root origin and are heard more easily. An early ES may merge with S_1 or, more likely, is thought by the examiner to be part of the S_1 complex (split S_1) (see Figure 5-1). In pulmonic stenosis, the more severe the valve obstruction is, the earlier the click; in these cases, the ES easily is confused with S_1.

Location

Aortic ejection sounds are audible at the cardiac base and the aortic area and, in particular, are heard well at the apex. In many individuals with an aortic ejection click, the sound is heard only at the apex. This is particularly true in the elderly or in patients with chronic lung disease. The systolic murmur of both aortic and pulmonary stenosis begins with the click, and this may obscure separate identification of the click at the base.

Pulmonic ejection sounds are heard best at the second and third left interspace and are heard poorly or inaudible at the apex. The pulmonic click of pulmonary hypertension also may be heard lower down the sternum. Respiratory variation, typical of valvular pulmonic stenosis, must be carefully sought; in more severe cases of pulmonic stenosis, the click occurs close to S_1 and may not be distinguished easily from it. A pulmonic click at the pulmonic area may easily be mistaken for S_1, which usually is quite soft at the left second or third interspace (see Figure 7-4). In patients suspected of having pulmonic stenosis, listen with the subject in an upright position; the resultant decrease in right ventricular venous return often results in the click becoming more audible both in inspiration and expiration.

Differential Diagnosis

Several possibilities may account for two discrete sounds heard in and about S_1: an S_4-S_1 combination, a split S_1, or an S_1 ejection click complex (see Figure 5-1). Loud systolic murmurs may contribute to the difficulty of identifying an ejection click by enveloping the discrete sound.

Table 7-1 lists differentiating features of the various diagnostic possibilities to be considered when two sounds are heard in rapid succession in the beginning of systole. Table 7-2 lists conditions associated with the different ejection sounds or clicks, some of which are discussed in the following sections.

Table 7-1. Differential Diagnosis of Systolic Ejection Sounds

Audible Sound Complex	Useful Differentiating Features
Aortic or pulmonic sound or click	Aortic: usually best heard at apex Pulmonic: inspiratory decrease common
	Evidence of associated aortic/pulmonary valve or root abnormality
	Firm pressure with stethoscope diaphragm increases audibility
S_4-S_1 complex	S_4 audibility enhanced with use of light pressure on stethoscope bell
	S_4 attenuates with firm pressure or use of stethoscope diaphragm
	S_4 not heard at cardiac base
	Often associated evidence of LV hypertrophy or dilatation
	S_4 waxes and wanes with changes in venous return
	RV S_4: will increase with inspiration; associated evidence for pulmonary hypertension or RV enlargement
Split S_1	Poor radiation of both components (M_1 and T_1) away from apex area
	Second component (T_1) usually not snappy or loud
	Second component (T_1) not audible at cardiac base
	Both components better heard with firm pressure on stethoscope diaphragm
Early click in mitral prolapse	Variable behavior of click timing with respect to body position, maneuvers
	Associated murmur of late systolic mitral regurgitation may be present, occasionally a holosystolic murmur

Table 7-2. Conditions Associated with Ejection Sound or Click

Condition
Aortic
Congenital valvular aortic stenosis
Bicuspid aortic valve
Aortic regurgitation
Aortic aneurysm
Aortic root dilatation
Systemic hypertension
Severe tetralogy of Fallot
Pulmonic
Pulmonary valve stenosis
Idiopathic dilatation of the pulmonary artery
Atrial septal defect
Chronic pulmonary hypertension
Tetralogy of Fallot (with pulmonic valve stenosis)
Pseudo-ejection sound
Prominent splitting of S_1
Increased T_1 (Ebstein's anomaly; ASD)
Hypertrophic cardiomyopathy
Early nonejection click of holosystolic mitral valve prolapse
High-pitched S_4 (S_1 confused for ES)

Aortic Stenosis

The presence of an ejection click strongly suggests the presence of a congenitally bicuspid aortic valve and, in general, excludes supra- or subvalvular stenosis or hypertrophic cardiomyopathy. Although an audible click indicates a valve with a significant degree of leaflet mobility, the presence or absence of an ES has no correlation with the severity of aortic stenosis. The intensity of A_2 usually parallels that of the aortic ejection click (see Figure 10-3).

Pulmonic Stenosis

Most patients with valvular pulmonic stenosis maintain a well-preserved pulmonary ES (see Figure 7-3). In very mild or very severe pulmonic stenosis, the click may be inaudible or, if present, inspiratory variation may be absent. The presence of a pulmonic click in a young patient with a prominent pulmonic outflow murmur and wide splitting of S_2 helps identify pulmonic stenosis; patients with an atrial septal defect usually have no prominent ejection sounds.

Aortic Root Dilatation

Ejection sounds may be heard whenever the central aorta is dilated. These sounds also may be detected in hypertensive patients. In the presence of an aortic ES, it may be difficult to exclude an associated aortic valve abnormality. Aortic root ES do not radiate well from the aortic area, whereas the ES of aortic valve disease often is heard best at the cardiac apex.

Pulmonary Hypertension

The presence of a pulmonic ejection click is common with chronic elevation of pulmonary artery pressure and may be a useful ancillary diagnostic sign of pulmonary hypertension, along with an increased P_2 and a right ventricular lift (see Figure 7-4).

Coarctation of Aorta

An aortic ejection click heard in a patient with aortic coarctation implies a coexisting, congenitally bicuspid aortic valve, a common associated abnormality (see Figure 7-1).

8

Heart Murmurs

Physicians must be able to assess heart murmurs accurately to properly evaluate patients with congenital or valvular heart disease. In the general population, systolic murmurs are widespread but reflect abnormal cardiac structure in only a small percentage of persons. The presence of a heart murmur raises questions regarding prophylaxis for endocarditis, restriction from athletics, eligibility for life insurance or employment, risk of pregnancy to the mother or fetus, and the safety of noncardiac surgery. In the practice of medicine, physicians confront these issues daily and must be able to distinguish heart murmurs in subjects who have no intrinsic cardiac abnormalities from those that indicate organic disease.

Significance of a Murmur

When someone is found to have a murmur, several issues require resolution. The first question to ask is whether the murmur is organic or pathologic or a normal variant. Based on the information derived from the cardiac physical examination, one can determine the likeliest hemodynamic cause of the murmur. Once the anatomic origin of an organic murmur is characterized, the possible etiologies of the heart disease should be investigated, and the severity of the underlying condition can be assessed.

Usually, a capable clinician can resolve these questions after a careful physical examination. While ancillary diagnostic testing (e.g., EKG, chest roentgenogram, M-mode or two-dimensional echocardiogram, cardiac catheterization) often is important, typically these studies provide additional data about the severity of a problem that already has been identified and roughly quantitated by the physical examination.

When a heart murmur is felt to be "innocent" (see Chapter 9), the diagnosis of *nondisease* should be made firmly and without equivocation. *Practical Point: Heart murmurs with no intrinsic cardiac abnormality are far more common than those with organic cardiovascular disease. Therefore, ruling out significant heart disease is an important aspect of everyday clinical practice.*

Physiology

Turbulence is the primary factor in the genesis of heart murmurs. Turbulent blood flow produces both physiologic and organic murmurs. An important determinant of turbulence is the velocity of blood flow: Increases in velocity result in marked increases in turbulence, often producing audible sound. An obstruction to blood flow, like stenosis, produces abnormal turbulence, which is related to both the velocity of blood flow and alterations in accelerating forces; turbulence increases as the gradient across the valve becomes larger. For any given size of valve orifice, an increase in blood flow results in increased flow velocity; conversely, for any given flow rate, a smaller or narrowing orifice results in a greater velocity of blood flow and a louder murmur.

Normal Ejection

During the first part of systole, there is a small pressure or "impulse" gradient between each ventricle and its respective great vessel (Figure 8-1), which may account for sufficient turbulence to produce cardiac sound.

Sound Frequency

In general, turbulent flow produces random sound that has many frequencies and results in mixed frequency murmurs. High flow rates or large gradients produce more high-pitched sound; low flow rates and small gradients produce low-pitched sound.

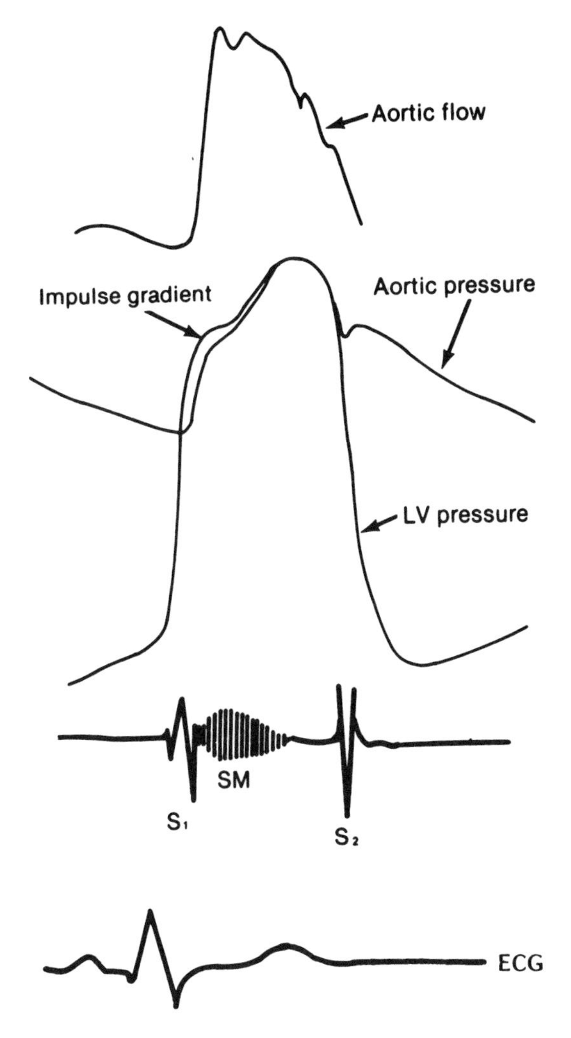

Figure 8-1. Pressure flow relationships of the systolic ejection or flow murmur. During early systole peak blood flow and velocity are maximal, producing sufficient turbulence for the production of audible sound. A typical systolic ejection murmur ends within the first two thirds of systole. Note the small "impulse gradient" in early systole.

Transmission

Transmission or radiation of cardiac sound results from vibration of cardiac structures and blood vessels set up by turbulence or eddy formation. High-frequency sound does not transmit well downstream. Low-frequency vibrations are heard better downstream and therefore transmit more widely.

General Principles of Cardiac Auscultation

Use of the Stethoscope

The bell of the stethoscope is ideal for low-frequency murmurs (25–125 cps) (see Figure 1-2); when the bell is used, light skin contact is desirable to maximize detection of low-pitched sound. The diaphragm is best for high-frequency or mixed-frequency murmurs; increasing pressure on the rigid diaphragm will attenuate lower-pitched sounds and accentuate the higher frequencies. One should routinely alter the stethoscope pressure during auscultation to assess optimally the frequency characteristics of heart sounds and murmurs.

Grading Murmurs

The 1 through 6 grading protocol was created to provide a systematic and consistent method of evaluating heart murmurs.

Grade 1. The faintest murmur that can be heard under optimal conditions (quiet room, relaxed patient and physician).

Grade 2. A soft but readily audible murmur.

Grade 3. A prominent murmur and always should stimulate a careful search for cardiac disease.

Grade 4. A very loud murmur that is palpable (thrill).

Grade 5. Louder still (thrill).

Grade 6. A murmur audible with the stethoscope held off the chest wall (thrill).

The intensity of a murmur is graded on a 1 to 6 basis (e.g., a 3/6 ejection murmur, a 2/6 decrescendo diastolic murmur). Most innocent or functional murmurs will be grade 1–2/6; some will be grade 3/6. Murmur grades of 5/6 or 6/6 are rare.

Valve Areas

Customarily, specific locations on the chest have been designated as relating to a particular cardiac valve. This practice stems from observations regarding the site where a specific murmur (e.g., aortic stenosis) usually is best heard. Therefore, the second right interspace is known as the *aortic area*; the second to third left interspace is the *pulmonary area*; the lower left sternal border is the *tricuspid area*; and the apex is the *mitral area*. However, there are many exceptions to this oversimplified approach. Radiation patterns of various organic murmurs often are discordant with the precise anatomic location of the valves that produce the murmur, making the specific precordial "area" less reliable in determining the site of origin of a murmur. Shah and Luisada have proposed the use of "areas" of auscultation relating to the underlying cardiac chambers (Table 8-1).

Classification of Heart Murmurs

The general classification of murmurs proposed by Aubrey Leatham in 1958 has been widely adopted (Table 8-2). Leatham divided systolic murmurs into two major types, *midsystolic ejection* and *pansystolic* or *regurgitant*. *Diastolic* and *continuous* murmurs are the other two major types of heart murmurs. Ejection murmurs not caused by valvular obstruction or narrowing are known as flow murmurs, functional murmurs, or innocent murmurs. When defining or classifying a murmur, it is desirable to use a physiologic descriptor as well as an indication of the timing of the murmur (e.g., late systolic regurgitant murmur or early systolic ejection murmur).

Systolic Murmurs

Ejection Murmurs

The most common murmur heard in everyday practice is the ejection or flow murmur produced by rapid ejection of blood during the first part of systole. Peak acceleration of blood flow occurs in early systole just after aortic valve opening. During the last third of systole very little forward flow occurs across the semilunar valves (see Figure 8-1). *Early systolic murmurs are common, even in the presence of normal valves and a basal cardiac output.* Irregular, thickened, or stenotic

Table 8-1. Locations of Auscultatory Sites

Area	Prior Designation	Location	Murmurs Heard Best	Sounds Heard
Left ventricular	"Mitral area"	At apex impulse: extends to 3–5 LICS, 2 cm medially and laterally to left anterior axillary line. Isolated LVE: extends medially; isolated RVE: may be displaced to left axilla	Mitral stenosis Mitral regurgitation Aortic stenosis Aortic insufficiency IHSS Functional middiastolic rumble	LV S_3 LV S_4 A_2
Right ventricular	"Tricuspid area"	Lower sternum and 3–5 LICS 2 cm to left and right Isolated RVE: can extend laterally and occupy the apex	Tricuspid stenosis Tricuspid regurgitation Pulmonary regurgitation Ventricular septal defect	RV S_3 RV S_4 TV opening snap
Left atrial		Left posterior thorax between axillary line and spine at level of scapular tip	Mitral regurgitation	
Right atrial		Lower sternum and 4–5 RICS, 2 cm to right of sternum	Tricuspid regurgitation	
Aortic area	"Erbs point" (third left interspace)	3 LICS near sternal edge across manubrium to 1–3 RICS, may include 2 LICS, suprasternal notch, right sternoclavicular joint	Aortic stenosis Aortic insufficiency Aortic flow murmurs	A_2 Aortic ejection click
Pulmonary area		1–3 LICS adjacent to sternum, medial left intraclavicular area; posterior thorax: T_{4-5} 2–3 cm to either side of spine	Pulmonary stenosis Pulmonary regurgitation Pulmonary flow murmurs PDA murmur	Pulmonary ejection click P_2
Descending thoracic aorta		Posterior thorax: $T_2 = T_{12}$, 2–3 cm to either side of the spine	Coarctation of the aorta Aortic aneurysms Aortic stenosis	

Table 8-2. Classification of Heart Murmurs

- Systolic
  - Ejection murmurs
    - Flow or functional murmurs
      - Innocent murmur
      - Physiologic murmur (related to increased cardiac output), such as due to anemia, thyrotoxicosis, or occurring after exercise
  - Pathologic or significant murmurs
    - Abnormal but nonstenotic aortic or pulmonary valve
    - Aortic or pulmonary valve stenosis
    - Dilatation of aorta or pulmonary artery
    - Left or right ventricular outflow tract obstruction (nonvalvular)
  - Regurgitant murmurs
    - Mitral regurgitation
    - Tricuspid regurgitation
    - Ventricular septal defect
- Diastolic
  - Semilunar valve incompetence
    - Aortic or pulmonary regurgitation
  - Ventricular filling murmurs
    - Mitral or tricuspid stenosis
    - Augmented AV valve flow (e.g., mitral regurgitation, VSD, ASD)
    - Presystolic murmur due to atrial contraction (e.g., mitral or tricuspid stenosis)
- Continuous
  - Communication between high pressure chamber or artery with low pressure chamber or vein (e.g., patent ductus arteriosus, coronary AV fistula, sinus of Valsalva to right atrial communication)

semilunar valve leaflets result in greater turbulence and increased murmur intensity.

The typical systolic ejection murmur begins after S_1 at the completion of isovolumic contraction (Figures 8-1, 8-2D, 8-3A). The classic flow murmur peaks early (crescendo), then falls away (decrescendo) as the velocity and the ejected volume of blood diminish in mid- to late systole. *The systolic ejection murmur usually ends before S_2.*

However, with semilunar valve stenosis, prolonged ventricular emptying may produce a late peaking murmur that can extend to or beyond A_2 or P_2. The intensity of the ejection murmur is related to the velocity of blood flow, which in turn is dependent on stroke volume, valve orifice area, and accelerating forces. A large stroke volume results in a louder and longer murmur.

Types of Ejection Murmurs

Murmurs related to the ejection of blood across the semilunar valves are either *flow related* or *pathologic* in origin. Some of their causes include

- Abnormal semilunar valve, no gradient.
- Abnormal semilunar valve, with gradient (stenosis).
- Increased diameter or dilatation of a great vessel.

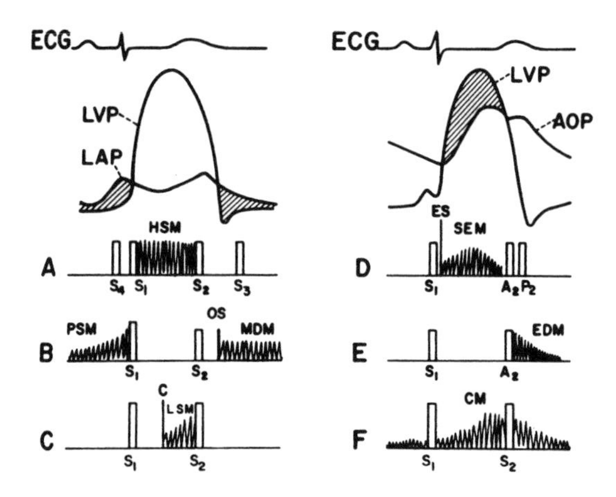

Figure 8-2. (A–F) Intracardiac pressures and heart murmurs in the major cardiac valve abnormalities. See the text for discussion of specific murmurs. LVP = left ventricular pressure, LAP = left atrial pressure, AOP = aortic pressure, HSM = holosystolic murmur, PSM = presystolic murmur, OS = opening snap, MDM = middiastolic murmur, C = midsystolic click, LSM = late-systolic murmur, ES = ejection sound, SEM = systolic ejection murmur, EDM = early-diastolic murmur, CM = continuous murmur. (Reprinted with permission from Crawford MH, O'Rourke RA. A systematic approach to the bedside differentiation of cardiac murmurs and abnormal sounds. *Curr Probl Cardiol.* 1979;1:1.)

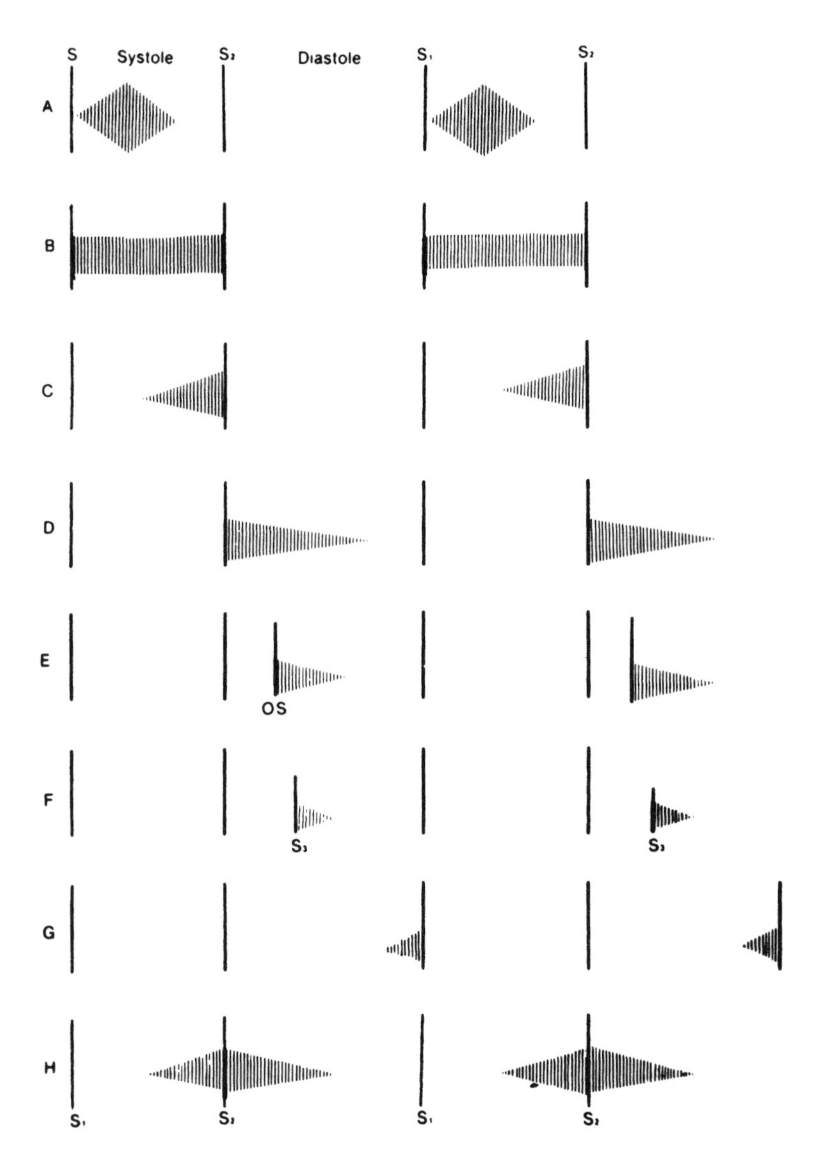

Figure 8-3. Major types of cardiac murmurs. See the text for description.

- Abnormal sub- or supravalvular narrowing of the left or right ventricular outflow tract.
- An abnormal increase in blood flow across a structurally normal outflow tract, where the augmented blood volume results from an underlying organic cardiac lesion (e.g., the systolic murmur associated with an atrial septal defect or pure aortic regurgitation).

Flow or Functional Murmur

Flow or functional murmurs are by far the most common heart murmurs and are found in many normal persons (see Chapter 9). In the presence of a normal resting cardiac output the murmur is known as an *innocent* or *functional murmur.* If the murmur is related to a hyperkinetic state with increased cardiac output and stroke volume, the murmur is known as a *physiologic murmur*.

Pathologic, Significant, or Organic Ejection Murmurs

Pathologic, significant, and organic ejection murmurs result from underlying structural abnormalities of the semilunar valves, the cardiac chambers, or great vessels. The causes are those of general ejection murmurs, as listed previously.

Systolic Regurgitant Murmurs

Systolic regurgitant murmurs are generated by a continuous systolic pressure gradient produced by an abnormal structural or functional communication between two chambers of the heart. A typical regurgitant murmur begins with the development of ventricular pressure (isovolumic contraction) and continues until S_2 (Figure 8-2A). If a large pressure gradient between two cardiac chambers persists into late systole, blood flow and cardiac sound will continue until the onset of diastole. The classic regurgitant murmur is holo- or pansystolic with a constant amplitude and shape throughout systole (Figures 8-2A and 8-3B). Systolic regurgitant murmurs are present in mitral and tricuspid regurgitation and ventricular septal defects. Late systolic murmurs, beginning after S_1 and extending to S_2, typically reflect mild degrees of mitral regurgitation (Figures 8-2C and 8-3C).

Diastolic Murmurs

Semilunar Valve Regurgitation

Semilunar valve regurgitation murmurs begin with semilunar valve closure (S_2) and usually are decrescendo in configuration (Figures 8-2E and 8-3D). The shape and length of the murmur reflect the diastolic pressure gradient between aorta or pulmonary artery and the respective ventricle. Because of the high velocity of regurgitant blood flow from the great vessels, the murmurs of semilunar valve incompetence typically are of high frequency.

Ventricular Filling Murmurs

A-V Valve Stenosis

A-V valve stenosis murmurs are caused by obstruction to inflow of blood to the left or right ventricle in patients with mitral or tricuspid valve stenosis (Figures 8-2B and 8-3E). The onset of the murmur follows complete opening of the A-V valve, and the murmur is middiastolic in timing. Typically, these murmurs are low pitched because of the relatively small pressure gradients between the atrium and ventricles, which result in low-flow velocity even with severe stenosis.

Increased A-V Valve Flow without Valvular Stenosis

Under conditions of excessive atrial blood volume and augmented flow across the mitral or tricuspid valve, a short, middiastolic "filling murmur" often can be heard. Such a murmur may begin with a ventricular filling sound (S_3; Figure 8-3F). Middiastolic flow murmurs are common when there is increased flow across an A-V valve due to a left-to-right shunt (atrial septal defect, ventricular septal defect, or patent ductus arteriosus). The Austin Flint murmur of aortic regurgitation is another variant of the "functional" diastolic filling murmur (see Chapter 12).

Presystolic Murmur

A late diastolic or presystolic murmur may be heard in patients with mild to moderate mitral or tricuspid stenosis; this results from augmentation of A-V flow following atrial contraction.

Continuous Murmurs

Continuous murmurs result from a persistent gradient between a high-pressure site (arterial or ventricular) and a low-pressure site (vein or right heart chamber). These murmurs typically begin in systole and "spill over" into early diastole, peaking in the mid- to late systole. Rarely, they are audible in late diastole (Figures 8-2F and 8-3H).

Diagnosis of Organic Murmurs

Because nonpathologic or innocent flow murmurs are so common, the clinician has a great responsibility to determine whether or not a heart murmur is pathologic. Chapter 9 discusses the characteristics of the innocent or physiologic ejection murmur. Unfortunately, only a few criteria absolutely identify the organic or pathologic cardiac murmur:

1. *All diastolic murmurs are pathologic.* No cardiac sound should be heard during diastole. Middiastolic flow murmurs across the mitral (VSD, PDA, mitral regurgitation) or tricuspid (ASD, tricuspid regurgitation) valves do not imply organic disease of the A-V valves but reflect the marked diastolic volume overload traversing the A-V valve during rapid ventricular filling.
2. *All pansystolic and late systolic murmurs are pathologic.* Cardiac sound typically is absent during the last third of ejection. Murmurs that extend to S_2 are organic and indicate continuing turbulent blood flow at a time when silence is expected. It is essential to listen selectively to late systole for the presence or absence of sound vibrations. In some varieties of mitral regurgitation, mitral regurgitant flow begins well after ejection, and abnormal blood flow into the left atrium occurs only during mid- to late systole (see Chapters 13 and 15). Therefore, a murmur beginning in the last third of systole usually reflects "late" mitral regurgitation.
3. *Continuous murmurs always indicate organic heart disease.* A murmur that continues up to S_2 and spills over into diastole must reflect a continuing pressure differential between two cardiovascular structures and is, therefore, abnormal.
4. *Very loud murmurs are usually pathologic.* Any murmur associated with a thrill (grade 4 or greater) has a pathologic basis. Table 8-3 lists common noncardiac conditions associated with an increase or decrease in murmur intensity. These factors always should be kept in mind during auscultation of the patient.
5. *Associated cardiac abnormalities raise the likelihood that a given heart murmur is organic.* For instance, the presence of left ventricular hypertrophy on precordial palpation, an ejection or midsystolic click, or an opening snap would suggest

Table 8-3. Factors Affecting the Loudness of Heart Murmurs

Increased intensity
High cardiac output (hyperdynamic) states
Thin chest wall
Narrow thoracic diameter; for example, "straight back," pectus excavatum
Anemia (decreased blood viscosity)
Tortuous aorta (close to chest wall)
Decreased intensity
Obesity
Muscular or thick chest wall
Obstructive lung disease
Barrel chest (increased A-P diameter)
Pericardial thickening or fluid
Decreased cardiac output (CHF, low ejection fraction)

that the heart murmur represents a cardiac structural abnormality. However, these phenomena may be unrelated to the production of the murmur itself.

6. *Frequency, shape* or *contour, and radiation characteristics of heart murmurs are too nonspecific to establish definitively the organic etiology of a murmur.*

Evaluation of Heart Murmurs

The clinician should take a systematic approach to the accurate assessment of heart murmurs. The following features of murmurs should be consciously analyzed in each patient:

- Whether the murmur is *systolic* or *diastolic.*
- The *timing* of the murmur within systole or diastole—early, mid, or late.
- The *duration* of the murmur.
- The *intensity* or *loudness* of the murmur; that is, its grade.

- The *transmission* of the murmur.
- The *frequency* and *shape* of the murmur.
- *Other cardiac abnormalities* present on examination that may relate to the etiology of the murmur.

Timing

Once it is clear that a given murmur is systolic or diastolic (see Chapter 1), it is necessary to clarify whether the murmur is early, mid, or late in systole or diastole.

Systole

All ejection murmurs, whether pathologic or not, are early to midsystolic in timing. A severe degree of obstruction to outflow will cause ejection murmurs to lengthen and peak later in systole. Not all early systolic murmurs are ejection murmurs. In some patients, the murmur of a ventricular septal defect or A-V valve regurgitation begins in early systole and tapers off in late systole, ending before A_2.

A "late-systolic murmur" is not heard in the first third of systole and should not be confused with an ejection murmur; latesystolic murmurs usually represent mitral regurgitation (see Figures 8-2C and 8-3C and Chapter 13). These murmurs begin in midsystole with sound vibrations heard up to A_2.

Diastole

Early-diastolic murmurs result from semilunar valve incompetence (aortic or pulmonary regurgitation). Middiastolic murmurs are produced by flow across either the mitral or tricuspid valve during passive filling of the ventricles. In stenosis of either A-V valve, the diastolic murmur is caused by a narrowed and obstructive orifice. Such murmurs lengthen in proportion to the severity of valvular obstruction, and cardiac sound may persist up to S_1. Middiastolic murmurs also can occur with no narrowing of the A-V valve if there is markedly augmented blood flow with rapid ventricular filling. Here, the murmur is brief and usually follows an S_3. Late-diastolic and presystolic murmurs are produced by atrial contraction in the presence of mitral or tricuspid stenosis (Figure 8-3G).

Continuous murmurs represent cardiac sound that spills over into diastole. Care must be taken to differentiate these murmurs from the combination of a long systolic and early diastolic murmur that can be heard in mixed semilunar valve stenosis and regurgitation.

Duration

Systole

The most important characteristic of systolic murmurs is their length. *Practical Point: Whether a systolic murmur extends to S_2 and, therefore, is holosystolic is the most valuable part of murmur analysis.* Any murmur that is truly holo- or pansystolic, regardless of shape, is caused by continuous pressure differential between two cardiac chambers (see Figure 8-2A). Therefore, the classic murmurs of a ventricular septal defect or mitral regurgitation (see Chapter 13) begin with S_1 and extend through S_2.

The presence of a long systolic murmur should stimulate a careful evaluation of late systole through selective listening. A careful focus on the last 25% of systole is important (Figure 8-4). If sound vibrations end before S_2, the murmur usually is an ejection murmur. If the murmur extends to S_2 (pansystolic), the differential diagnosis should include regurgitant lesions as well as severe semilunar valvular stenosis.

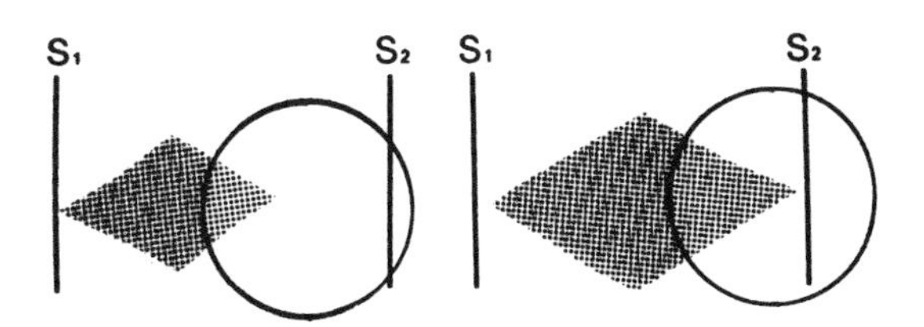

Figure 8-4. The importance of late systole in evaluation of systolic murmurs. It is essential to assess the last part of systole to determine whether a murmur is ejection in nature or holosystolic. On the left, an early peaking murmur ends before the last third of systole. This is the rule in functional murmurs or with mild semilunar valve stenosis. On the right, a long ejection murmur is shown that peaks later in systole. Sound vibrations extend to S_2, suggesting severe obstruction to ventricular outflow. In severe semilunar valve stenosis, the vibrations may extend beyond S_2.

Diastole

The duration of diastolic murmurs is important, particularly in the assessment of left ventricular filling murmurs. As already emphasized, flow across a nonobstructive or mildly stenotic A-V valve produces a short middiastolic murmur. A long diastolic murmur following an opening snap is indicative of a persistent A-V gradient and significant mitral stenosis. With short cycle lengths, these murmurs extend to S_1.

Murmurs of semilunar valve regurgitation usually are quite long and may be pandiastolic, continuing to S_1. Usually, these high-frequency murmurs are of low intensity and may be very faint in late diastole. With severe aortic regurgitation, particularly in acute valvular incompetence, the exceedingly high left-ventricular end-diastolic pressure may produce a small or absent aortic left-ventricular gradient in late diastole, resulting in a relatively short diastolic regurgitant murmur (see Chapter 12).

Intensity

The intensity, or loudness, of a murmur is directly related to the degree of turbulence. Increased volume or velocity of flow results in enhanced turbulence and louder murmurs.

Often, it is assumed that the intensity of a murmur is directly related to the severity of the underlying condition. Although this is frequently true, there are many exceptions. The careful auscultator should be aware of the various factors that may modify the intensity of murmurs (see Table 8-3). The common causes of decreased intensity of heart murmurs include poor cardiac function that results in a reduced stroke volume and ejection velocity and "buffering" of the heart from the stethoscope by excessive body tissue (e.g., obstructive lung disease, obesity). For example, in congestive heart failure resulting from aortic stenosis or mitral regurgitation, the systolic murmur may be soft and unimpressive, possibly causing a false assessment of the underlying problem. On the other hand, occasional innocent murmurs may be prominent (but never of grade 4/6 intensity). The classic, small ventricular septal defect can produce an extremely loud murmur.

Transmission

Radiation and transmission patterns of murmurs are directly related to the intensity, or loudness, of the murmur. Loud murmurs transmit widely; soft ones do not. High-frequency sound is heard best proximal or "upstream" from the origin of the murmur; low-frequency vibrations transmit best "downstream" or distal to the murmur's origin. This accounts for the common observation that the harsh components of the aortic stenosis murmur transmit to the base and neck, while higher frequency vibrations are best heard at the apex.

The cardiac auscultatory regions (see Table 8-1) are related to the typical radiation patterns of classic valvular defects.

Shape

Assessing the contour or shape of heart murmurs may help the clinician distinguish systolic ejection murmurs (crescendo-decrescendo) from regurgitant (holosystolic) ones. Recordings of murmurs using selected frequency filters may be different from what actually is heard by the human ear. The typical kite-shaped or diamond-shaped ejection murmur often looks far more classic on a phonocardiogram than it appears to the ear, which may perceive only a rough, slightly tapering murmur ending before S_1. The true shape of a murmur is more difficult to determine than is commonly appreciated.

There are important exceptions to the classic contour of murmurs. For example, the pansystolic murmur of mitral regurgitation may have late systolic accentuation or can taper off in late systole. It is useful to diagram the shape of the murmur in the clinical record.

Frequency

The pitch, or frequency, of a heart murmur has some diagnostic value and should be noted. Table 8-4 lists the range of frequencies for most cardiac murmurs. Because of a large proportion of dominant higher frequencies, higher-pitched murmurs are more musical or pure in tone than lower-frequency ones. These often are called *blowing* murmurs. Very harsh murmurs (e.g., aortic valve stenosis) are mixtures of medium and high frequencies; the ear best perceives the lower tones, which tend to mask the higher frequencies. Murmurs with a preponderance of a particular frequency often have a certain resonance that is called *musical* or *vibratory*. Murmurs with a relatively clear pitch and pure fundamental tone often are called *cooing* or *seagull* murmurs.

Table 8-4. Frequency and Pitch of Common Cardiac Murmurs

	cps	Common Descriptive Terms	Examples
Low frequency	25–125	Rumbling, low pitched	Diastolic murmur of mitral stenosis
Medium frequency	125–300	Rough "flow" murmur	Innocent murmur, physiologic flow murmur
High frequency	>300	Blowing, whirring, high pitched	Aortic regurgitation, mitral regurtitation

9

The Systolic Ejection Murmur: Innocent, Physiologic, and Pathologic

A variety of normal and abnormal conditions can produce the relatively nonspecific "ejection" murmur. Most systolic murmurs heard in everyday practice are related to physiologic blood flow and of no clinical importance. It is imperative for the physician to properly identify these murmurs, thus avoiding the need for referral to a cardiologist, additional diagnostic tests, prophylaxis against acute rheumatic fever and bacterial endocarditis, and restriction of activities or employment.

Innocent or Functional Murmurs

The innocent murmur, by far the most common murmur heard in clinical practice, has certain characteristics that should enable the careful examiner to identify it accurately more than 90% of the time. If ancillary techniques also are employed (ECG, chest roentgenogram, and occasionally, echocardiography), virtually all functional systolic ejection murmurs can be properly classified.

Terminology

There are actually dozens of names for the innocent systolic murmur. Some examples include *Still's murmur, normal murmur, harmless murmur, innocuous murmur, basal ejection murmur, twanging string murmur, nonorganic murmur,* and *vibratory murmur. The sine qua non is that the underlying cardiovascular system is entirely normal and the murmur is audible at rest.*

The use of such descriptive terms as *flow, innocent,* or *functional murmur* is important, as it clearly implies that a systolic ejection murmur is not the result of an organic valve lesion or an abnormal communication within the heart or great vessels. Another commonly used term for such murmurs is *physiologic*, implying that the murmur results from blood flow and turbulence produced by normal cardiac structures. *Innocent* and *benign* are commonly employed terms, indicating a normal functional heart murmur audible under basal conditions. When such murmurs become louder with exercise, excitement, anemia, or tachycardia, they may be labeled *physiologic murmurs.*

Etiology

Innocent or physiologic murmurs are due to rapid early ejection of blood into the aorta, producing sufficient turbulence to yield an audible sound. Studies in children suggest that enhanced cardiac contractility is an important common denominator in the genesis of an innocent murmur, particularly if the murmur persists through childhood.

Age and Incidence

Under optimal acoustic conditions, experienced clinicians hear sound vibrations in systole in as many as 80–90% of children and young adults. The majority of these subjects will have an audible S_3 as well (Figure 9-1). With increasing age, the innocent murmur tends to attenuate or disappear; nevertheless, it is common (30–40% of individuals) to hear a soft systolic ejection murmur in normal adults.

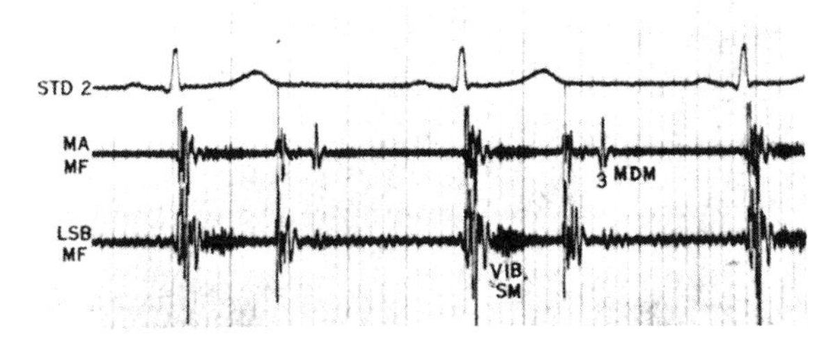

Figure 9-1. Functional systolic ejection murmur and third heart sound in a normal child. Note the short vibratory systolic murmur and the prominent S_3 (3) followed by a brief low-intensity middiastolic murmur (MDM). MA = mitral area, MF = medium frequency, LSB = left sternal border. (Reprinted with permission from McLaren MJ et al. Innocent murmurs and third heart sounds in black school children. *Br Heart J*. 1980;43:67.)

Systolic Murmur of Aging

Many older subjects in the sixth through ninth decades have an audible systolic ejection murmur that may have a different etiology than the innocent murmur of youth. These murmurs typically radiate well to the aortic area (second right interspace) and neck and also may be heard well at the apex. They often have a rougher quality than the typical innocent murmur of childhood and are particularly common in patients with hypertension. These systolic murmurs reflect underlying aortic valve sclerosis; they can simulate valvular aortic stenosis and, on occasion, may present a difficult differential problem. When accompanied by ECG changes or cardiovascular symptoms, it is easy to confuse these murmurs with those reflecting organic heart disease. Particular attention should be paid to the carotid pulse for signs of aortic stenosis, although this can be misleading because of age-related compliance changes in the peripheral vessels (see Chapter 2). The length of the systolic murmur also is useful in assessing whether the murmur is significant. If the murmur ends well before S_2, important aortic valve stenosis is unlikely. *Practical Point: Echocardiography should be employed in doubtful cases to assess the thickness and excursion of the aortic valve cusps.*

Location, Loudness, and Radiation

The innocent murmur is best heard along the left sternal border at the second to fourth interspace, most often between the apex and lower sternal border. Both the pulmonic and aortic valves are located in this region; it is important to assess the site of maximal intensity of the murmur. Innocent murmurs are uncommonly loudest at the apex. As a rule, they do not radiate well into the neck, although loud flow murmurs easily may be heard throughout the precordium. Some innocent murmurs radiate into the carotid arteries. Normal flow murmurs typically are of low or moderate intensity (usually 1–2/6) and never of grade 4/6 intensity. Thin persons tend to have louder innocent murmurs; a particularly loud systolic murmur in a subject who is very muscular, barrel chested, or obese should prompt a careful search for organic disease.

Length, Shape, and Quality

The typical innocent murmur occupies less than two thirds of systole and is crescendo-decrescendo in configuration (see Figures 8-1, 8-2, 8-3A, and 9-1). The murmur usually is of low to medium frequency (60–180 Hz) and often has a preponderance of relatively pure frequencies. It may appear to be vibratory to the ear; terms such as *whirring, buzzing*, and *humming* are not uncommon descriptors.

Response to Maneuvers

The intensity, or loudness, of an innocent or flow murmur is enhanced by anything that increases the velocity of blood flow. Exertion, anxiety, or excitement exaggerates this murmur. Sitting or standing usually attenuates the innocent murmur by reducing the cardiac output. The typical functional murmur may become much softer or even disappear when the patient is in the upright position.

Associated Findings

The presence of an accompanying cardiovascular abnormality makes the diagnosis of an innocent murmur more tenuous. For example, a coexisting systolic ejection or nonejection click, diastolic murmur, opening snap, or left ventricular heave indicates a probable cardiac abnormality. Nevertheless, such finding may exist in association with an unrelated innocent murmur.

The following are some associated physical findings that suggest a systolic ejection murmur may not be innocent:

- Ejection sound
- Audible expiratory splitting of S_2
- Fixed splitting of S_2
- Mid- or late-systolic click
- Opening snap
- Diastolic murmur
- Very loud S_1
- Hyperdynamic or sustained left ventricular impulse
- Right ventricular heave
- Very loud A_2 or P_2

The characteristics of S_2 are useful in evaluation of a systolic ejection murmur. Completely normal splitting of S_2 makes an ASD or pulmonic stenosis most unlikely. In suspicious cases, a full cardiac evaluation is necessary, including an EKG and an echocardiogram.

Physiologic Murmurs

The distinction between an innocent murmur and a physiologic flow murmur is that the latter is caused by a *transient increase* in blood volume or velocity of ejection. When the causative factor for the augmented blood flow is removed (e.g., correction of anemia, lysis of fever, childbirth), the murmur no longer is audible or there is only a faint (grade 1–2/6) innocent murmur.

Pathologic or Abnormal Ejection Murmurs

Systolic Ejection Murmurs Caused by Abnormalities of the Cardiovascular System

In certain situations, underlying cardiac disease results in an increased cardiac stroke volume that produces a flow murmur; in these cases, the structural abnormality may be only indirectly related to the murmur. For example, in atrial septal defects, the augmented blood flow produced by the large left-to-right shunt produces a systolic ejection murmur in the second to third left interspace. This is an example of pulmonary artery origin of a flow murmur. In aortic or pulmonary regurgitation, the ventricles eject an abnormally large stroke volume into their respective great vessels, and a systolic flow murmur characteristically is present. In severe aortic regurgitation, the associated systolic murmur can be very loud (grade 3 to 4) with no valve stenosis: The deformed aortic valve leaflets often are abnormal and contribute to the turbulent blood flow resulting in a systolic murmur.

Abnormal Semilunar Valves

The classic organic systolic ejection murmur is that of aortic or pulmonic valve stenosis (see Chapter 10). A reduction of valve orifice area to at least 60–70% of normal is required before there is pressure difference across the valve in the resting state; mildly fused or rigid cusps may not produce sufficient obstruction to result in a pressure gradient. It may be impossible to diagnose early or mild aortic valve stenosis at the bedside. The presence or absence of an ejection click, abnormal S_2, delayed or small volume carotid pulse, palpable left ventricular hypertrophy, or echocardiographic abnormalities all help in the differential diagnosis of an innocent flow murmur versus mild valvular stenosis.

In general, the more significant is the valve stenosis, the later the peaking and the longer the murmur (see Chapter 10). The gap between the end of the sound vibrations and S_2 narrows with increasing obstruction of either the aortic or pulmonary valve. Other associated abnormalities (abnormal precordial motion, S_4, ejection click, abnormal splitting of S_2) are likely to be prominent with increasing grades of obstruction.

Hypertrophic Cardiomyopathy

Hypertrophic cardiomyopathy, a condition in which there is abnormal muscular thickening of the interventricular septum and an abnormal relation of the anterior leaflet of the mitral valve, produces variable obstruction to left ventricular ejection (see Chapter 11). A long systolic ejection murmur is the hallmark of hypertrophic cardiomyopathy. Even in subjects with no measurable gradient, a murmur usually is present.

In hypertrophic cardiomyopathy, the maximum intensity of the murmur usually is heard lower on the chest than in valvar aortic stenosis, and its location is more medial than the typical mitral regurgitation murmur. The presence of a brisk carotid pulse, a double precordial LV impulse, and a loud S_4 is strong evidence for hypertrophic cardiomyopathy (see Chapter 11).

Other Causes of Systolic Ejection Murmurs

Coarctation of Aorta

A systolic ejection murmur usually is present in patients with coarctation. Its site of maximal intensity (left posterior thorax) and timing (beginning well after S_1, often spilling over into diastole) are important clues. Many patients with this disorder have an associated congenital bicuspid aortic valve, which results in a systolic ejection click and an early systolic ejection murmur at the base (see Chapters 7 and 10). The cardinal diagnostic feature of coarctation is the finding of delayed and diminished femoral artery pulsations.

Mitral Regurgitation

The spectrum of murmurs found in mitral regurgitation is wide (see Chapters 13 and 15). On occasion, the murmur may taper off in late systol; and in others, it takes on a crescendo-decrescendo configuration. This is an uncommon finding in rheumatic mitral regurgitation and more likely to be found in the unusual etiologies of mitral regurgitation, such as hypertrophic cardiomyopathy, mitral prosthetic valve dysfunction, ruptured chordae tendinae, and papillary muscle dysfunction.

Part II

Physical Findings in Specific Cardiovascular Conditions

10

Aortic Stenosis

Valvular aortic stenosis has three major causes: congenital, rheumatic, and degenerative. Aortic stenosis is a valve lesion in which the physical findings are directly related to the underlying hemodynamic burden.

Etiology

The majority of cases of isolated aortic stenosis in patients under 50 years of age is due to a congenital defect, usually a bicuspid aortic valve. This anomaly is perhaps the most common congenital cardiac abnormality, estimated to occur in 1–2% of the general population. Many persons with this lesion have a structural abnormality of the valve (audible ejection click with or without a short systolic murmur) but show no evidence of obstruction to blood flow. In patients with coexistent mitral valve disease with or without a prior history of acute rheumatic fever, rheumatic heart disease is the likely cause of aortic stenosis. In older adults with isolated aortic stenosis but no evidence of other valve involvement, the most common etiology is degenerative stiffening and thickening of the leaflets of an inherently normal tricuspid aortic valve. Calcification often occurs, leading to a further reduction in orifice area (Figure 10-1A).

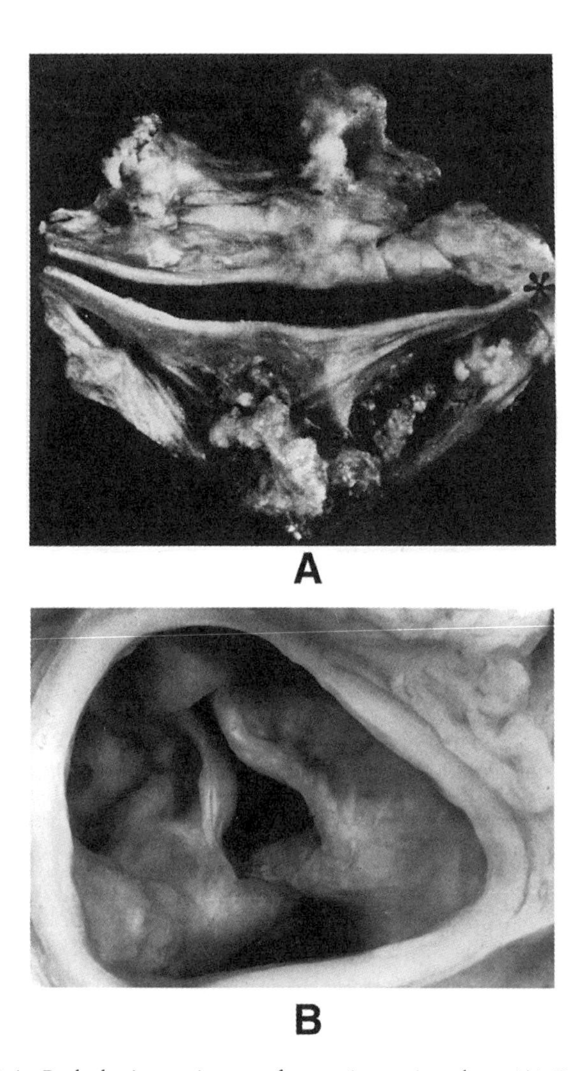

Figure 10-1. Pathologic specimens of stenotic aortic valves. (A) Congenitally bicuspid valve with calcification in valve pockets and mild fusion of the right commissure (*). (B) Postrheumatic aortic stenosis, in which there is an eccentric commissural lesion of all three commissures with heavy calcification. (A: Reprinted with permission from Subramanian R, Olson LG, Edwards WD. Surgical pathology of pure aortic stenosis; a study of 374 cases. *Mayo Clin Proc.* 1984;59:683. B: Reprinted with permission from Becker AE, Anderson RH. *Cardiac Pathology.* New York: Raven Press; 1983.)

Frequently, older persons, especially those with hypertension, develop nonobstructive thickening of the base of the aortic valve cusps. Known as *aortic sclerosis*, this is the most common cause of a systolic murmur in the elderly population. This murmur can simulate obstructive aortic stenosis, and it is important to differentiate the two entities (see later).

Pathophysiology

The normal aortic valve area in adults ranges between 2.5 and 3.5 cm^2. The valve has three cusps or leaflets of equal size. Reduction of the size of the aortic orifice does not result in a pressure drop across the valve at rest until at least 50% of the valve area is narrowed (i.e., aortic valve area of approximately 1.5 cm^2). However, a prominent systolic murmur may be present even in mild degrees of aortic stenosis. As the aortic orifice narrows, left ventricular pressure becomes further elevated to maintain forward blood flow and a normal systemic arterial pressure. Hemodynamically significant aortic stenosis occurs when the aortic valve area is reduced by 60–75%, resulting in a calculated aortic valve area of 0.7–0.8 cm^2 (Figure 10-1B). Symptoms are likely to appear at this stage, and evidence for left ventricular hypertrophy is usually present. Moderate aortic stenosis is present when the peak systolic left ventricular-aortic gradient is 50–60 mmHg. Severe aortic stenosis is present when the gradient is 75–80 mmHg or higher, assuming a normal stroke volume. The onset of left ventricular dysfunction and congestive heart failure may lower substantially the peak-to-peak systolic gradient.

In aortic stenosis the left ventricle undergoes concentric hypertrophy; this process produces a thick-walled chamber with no dilatation of the LV cavity. *Practical Point: Severe left ventricular dilatation and enlargement, as detected by palpation, chest roentgenogram, or echocardiography, is not a characteristic of compensated, pure aortic stenosis.*

Left ventricular systolic pressure must increase markedly to maintain adequate flow across a severely obstructed valve. With long-standing aortic stenosis, left ventricular contractile force is reduced. When this occurs, the heart usually dilates and symptoms of congestive heart failure develop. Paradoxically, the physical findings of aortic stenosis may become *less impressive* with the onset of left ventricular dilatation and congestive heart failure.

Physical Examination

Blood Pressure

In the absence of hypertension or associated aortic regurgitation, systolic blood pressure is normal in most subjects with aortic stenosis. With advanced degrees of aortic obstruction, the pulse pressure narrows as systolic arterial pressure decreases.

Contrary to popular belief, systemic arterial *hypertension* can be associated with significant valvular aortic stenosis, particularly in the older population. Systolic pressures greater than 140 mmHg often are found in older subjects with aortic stenosis.

Carotid Arterial Pulse

A hallmark of aortic stenosis is the typical slow-rising, small-volume arterial pulse (Figures 2-3, 10-2, and 10-3, and Table 10-1). Usually, there is an associated systolic thrill or shudder on the upstroke of the pulse. The classic pulse in aortic stenosis often is called *pulsus parvus et tardus* (slow and late pulse) or an *anacrotic* pulse. *Practical Point: The classic carotid pulse in aortic stenosis has a slowed upstroke, reduced amplitude, and sustained contour, with or without an accompanying palpable thrill.*

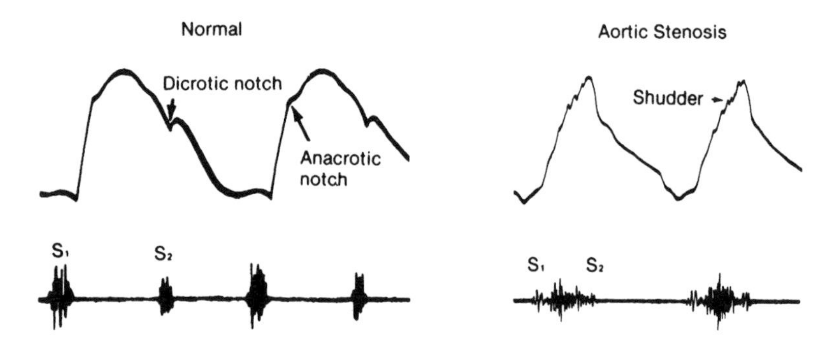

Figure 10-2. Carotid arterial pulse in aortic stenosis. (Left) A diagram of the normal carotid contour. (Right) A carotid pulse tracing from a patient with significant valvular aortic stenosis. Note the delayed upstroke and shudder that represents the transmitted murmur. The pulse volume usually is diminished in aortic stenosis (pulsus parvus et tardus).

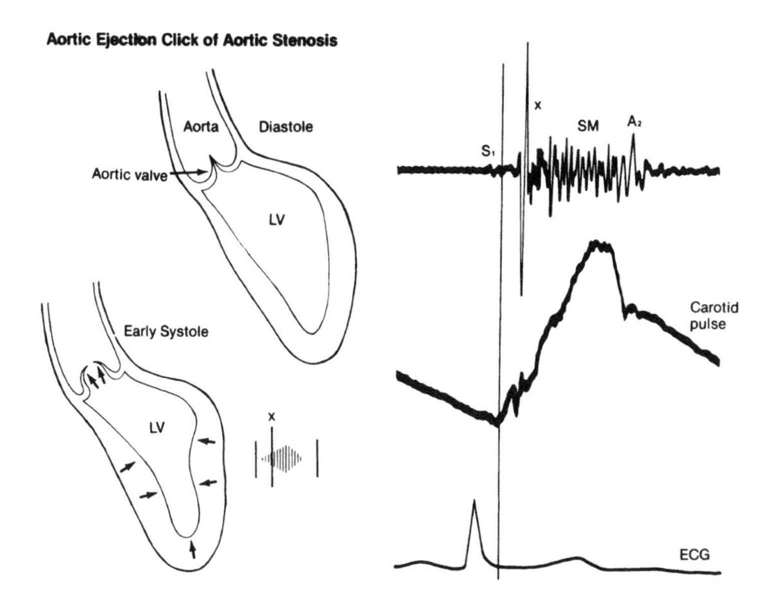

Figure 10-3. Ejection click associated with aortic stenosis due to a congenitally bicuspid valve. Note the high-frequency, high-amplitude sound that follows S_1 and is coincident with the onset of ejection into the aorta. The aortic ejection sound is formed by sudden cessation of the opening motion of the abnormal valve leaflets (doming). Note also the delayed carotid upstroke and long systolic murmur.

Table 10-1. Cardinal Features of the Carotid Pulse in Valvular Aortic Stenosis

Slow rising (pulsus parvus)
Delayed peak (pulsus tardus or plateau pulse)
Small volume
Palpable thrill
Prominent anacrotic notch (usually not palpable)

In detecting aortic stenosis, the focus of the examination of the arterial system should be on the carotid arteries and not on the peripheral pulses. The normal alterations of increased amplitude of the arterial pulse wave contour in the peripheral circulation minimizes the diagnostic usefulness of the brachial or radial arteries (see Figure 2-2).

Severity

The severity of the valvular obstruction is roughly proportional to the degree of abnormality of the carotid pulse in younger subjects. Unfortunately, many factors may affect the pulse contour, and it is not uncommon to seriously under- or overestimate the severity of aortic stenosis by carotid artery palpation (Table 10-2). *Practical Point: In an adult under 60 years of age with clinically normal left ventricular function (no congestive heart failure or gross cardiomegaly), a completely normal carotid pulse contour and arterial pulse pressure generally excludes moderate to severe aortic stenosis.* A distinctly delayed carotid upstroke in the same setting is consistent with moderate to severe valve obstruction.

Factors Leading to Underestimation of Severity of Aortic Stenosis from Carotid Pulse Analysis

Table 10-2 lists factors or associated conditions that may mask the severity of aortic stenosis (see also Chapter 2). In children with congenital aortic stenosis, the arterial pulse may be only mildly deranged or even normal in the face of a large aortic valve gradient, due to a highly elastic and compliant peripheral vasculature. A common problem in older adults is the *loss of arterial elasticity* that occurs with aging, with or without associated systolic hypertension. In this setting, a normal or reduced stroke volume ejected across the stenotic valve may *not* produce the typical slow-upstroke, small-volume pulse of

Table 10-2. Pitfalls in Evaluating the Arterial Pulse in Aortic Stenosis

Factors that can "normalize" the arterial pulse and mask the apparent severity
High cardiac output and elastic vessels in children and young patients
Increased stiffness of vessels in the elderly
Associated aortic regurgitation
Systemic hypertension
Low stroke volume of congestive heart failure
Factors that can exaggerate the apparent severity of aortic stenosis
Decreased left ventricular function
Hypovolemia
Mitral stenosis

aortic stenosis because of the decreased compliance of the systemic arteries. Therefore, a "normal" rate of rise and pulse amplitude will be misleading in this setting.

Aortic regurgitation, a frequent accompaniment of aortic stenosis, may have an important effect on the arterial pulse of aortic stenosis. The increased stroke volume and rate of ejection in aortic regurgitation may result in a carotid upstroke with a fuller pulse volume and a greater rate of rise than found in an equivalent degree of aortic stenosis without regurgitation.

Jugular Venous Pulse

The venous pulse configuration and pressure are unremarkable in aortic stenosis. Occasionally, the jugular A wave will be prominent in the absence of an elevation in mean jugular pressure. If biventricular heart failure is present, the mean jugular pressure will be elevated.

Precordial Motion

The apex impulse in hemodynamically important, compensated aortic stenosis typically is a *sustained* left ventricular lift with little or no leftward displacement of the point of maximal impulse (PMI) (Figure 10-4). The duration and force of the left ventricular impulse is increased due to the increased left ventricular mass, high intraventricular pressure, and obstruction to ventricular outflow.

A normal LV impulse is characteristic of mild aortic stenosis; in subjects with lung disease, obesity, deep chests, or large breasts, the apex beat may be diminutive or impalpable even in the presence of severe aortic stenosis. The presence of a sustained but otherwise unimpressive left ventricular impulse in an older subject with a large chest and a long systolic murmur suggests important aortic obstruction. *Practical Point: The concentrically hypertrophied left ventricle of isolated aortic stenosis does not produce significant lateral or downward displacement unless cardiac dilatation has occurred or there is associated aortic regurgitation.* During precordial palpation, pay close attention to the *duration* of the apex impulse, which will be sustained into the second half of systole in significant aortic valve obstruction (see Chapter 4).

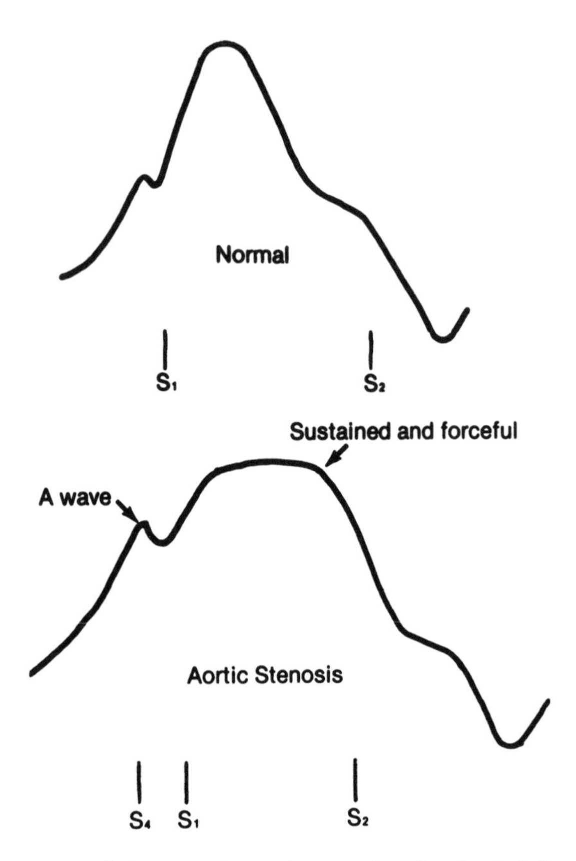

Figure 10-4. Precordial motion in aortic stenosis. The classic left ventricular impulse in left ventricular pressure overload due to aortic stenosis is concentric hypertrophy with no left ventricular dilatation, producing a sustained impulse that remains palpable into late systole. The impulse typically is more forceful than normal. Careful palpation frequently will detect a palpable A wave (S_4).

A palpable A wave (presystolic distention of the left ventricle) in the supine or left decubitus position is a most valuable observation (see Figures 6-2 and 10-4). This finding indicates elevation of left ventricular end-diastolic pressure and suggests a thick, noncompliant chamber; in younger subjects (e.g., <60 years old), it suggests a clinically significant aortic valve gradient.

Systolic Thrill

The loud, harsh (grade 3–4/6) murmur of aortic stenosis often is accompanied by a systolic thrill. The most common location of the thrill is the first or second right intercostal space, with radiation upward and rightward toward the neck and right shoulder. *Practical Point: For optimal detection of the systolic thrill, ask the subject to sit up and lean forward while holding his or her breath in expiration.*

A systolic thrill is the rule, not the exception, in aortic stenosis. Detection of a thrill indicates that aortic stenosis is present but does not necessarily indicate severe obstruction.

Heart Sounds

First Heart Sound

The first heart sound usually is unremarkable in isolated aortic stenosis. It may be decreased in intensity but never accentuated. A loud "S_1" in a patient with suspected or proven aortic stenosis suggests the presence of an aortic ejection sound or associated mitral stenosis.

Second Heart Sound

Because abnormalities in the amplitude of A_2 and the inspiratory behavior of S_2 are common in aortic stenosis, careful assessment of S_2 is particularly useful.

Intensity of A_2

In patients with pliable and relatively thin aortic leaflets, A_2 may be normal or even increased in amplitude. This is typical of congenital aortic stenosis (bicuspid valve) without calcification and occasionally may be found in young subjects with severe aortic obstruction. However, as thickening and rigidity of the aortic leaflets ensues, the amplitude of A_2 decreases. Calcification of the valve usually contributes to the diminished loudness of A_2. A_2 may be totally inaudible in severe aortic stenosis. *Practical Point: The amplitude of the aortic ejection click and that of A_2 are closely related. Both are prominent in a subject with a pliable, noncalcified bicuspid valve. Both are decreased in intensity in the presence of calcium or significant valvular thickening.*

Because A_2 commonly is soft or absent in aortic stenosis, a normal or increased P_2 (e.g., as might occur with associated pulmonary hypertension or congestive heart failure) can readily be mistaken for A_2.

Splitting of S_2 in Aortic Stenosis
Hemodynamically important aortic stenosis produces abnormalities in the sequence of S_2 splitting (Figure 10-5). The characteristic alteration of S_2 is an increase in the Q-A_2 interval with A_2 "moving into P_2" and a tendency for S_2 to become single. If LV ejection time is delayed substantially, reversed or paradoxic splitting of S_2 occurs (see Chapter 5 and Figures 5-3 and 10-5). *Practical Point: Detection of paradoxic splitting of S_2 in aortic stenosis in the absence of left bundle branch block or impaired left ventricular function is an important observation that implies that the left ventricular-aortic gradient is 75 mmHg or greater, such as in severe aortic stenosis.*

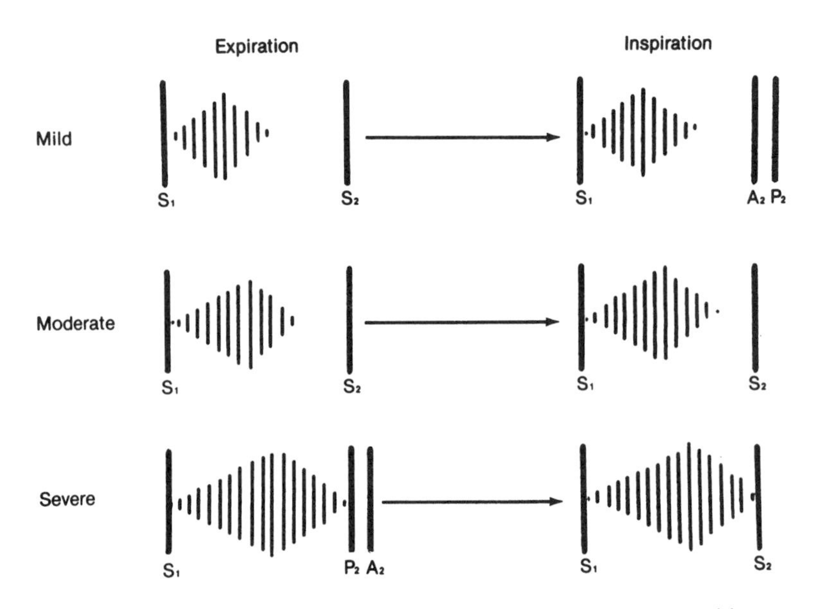

Figure 10-5. Patterns of S_2 splitting in aortic stenosis. (Upper) In mild degrees of left ventricular obstruction splitting of S_2 remains physiologic. (Middle) Frequently, a single S_2 is heard in aortic stenosis, reflecting moderate obstruction; the delayed A_2 results in fusion of the two components of S_2. Marked attenuation in the intensity of A_2 from severe fibrocalcific changes may cause A_2 to be inaudible and result in a single S_2 (which actually is P_2). (Lower) With advanced aortic stenosis, left ventricular ejection time is prolonged sufficiently that, in expiration, aortic valve closure follows pulmonic closure. During inspiration, P_2 moves away from S_1 and may become synchronous with A_2, resulting in paradoxic or reversed splitting of S_2. Note the increasing length and time to peak intensity of the murmur with increasing severity of obstruction.

Normal splitting of S_2 generally is found in mild aortic stenosis in adults (see Figure 10-5) and is common in congenital aortic stenosis, even when severe. A single S_2 also may result from a decreased intensity of A_2 due to fibrocalcific changes. *Practical Point: In approximately two thirds of older patients with moderate to severe aortic stenosis, S_2 will be single. S_2 will be reversed or paradoxic in another 20–25% and completely normal in a small number of patients.*

Third Heart Sound

An S_3 is not a normal or expected finding in adults with aortic stenosis. Its presence suggests significant left ventricular dysfunction or overt congestive heart failure. When an S_3 is heard, look for evidence of left ventricular dilatation as well as pulsus alternans. In such cases, the left ventricular impulse often will be displaced laterally. Remember that an S_3 is a normal finding in children and young adults.

Fourth Heart Sound

An S_4 is a valuable clue to the presence of LV hypertrophy and decreased LV compliance associated with severe aortic stenosis but only in younger patients (e.g., age 12–40). The presence of an audible or palpable S_4 correlates with a large left ventricular aortic gradient (greater than 70 mmHg) and abnormally elevated left ventricular end-diastolic pressure (LVEDP). Because an S_4 may be normal in young children and commonly found in older patients with coexisting atherosclerotic heart disease or hypertension, its significance is considerably reduced in these age groups. *Practical Point: The presence of an audible S_4 in an older patient does not necessarily mean the aortic stenosis is severe.* The finding of a *palpable* S_4 (presystolic distention) *at any age* (see Figure 10-4) in a patient with aortic stenosis implies that the valve obstruction is of major hemodynamic importance.

Aortic Ejection Click

The detection of an aortic ejection click (see Chapter 7) or sound is an important observation (see Figure 10-3):

1. It confirms the diagnosis of structural heart disease in a patient with a systolic ejection murmur.
2. It localizes the abnormality to the aortic valve (in the absence of a dilated aorta or chronic hypertension).

3. It suggests that the etiology of the valve abnormality is a congenitally deformed aortic valve, usually a bicuspid valve.

Practical Point: Although an ejection click indicates that the deformity is at aortic valve level, its presence does not correlate with the severity of the lesion.

The ejection click is related to the maximal upward excursion of an abnormal bicuspid or unicuspid valve (see Figure 10-1), occurring precisely when the pistonlike upward motion of the valve leaflets abruptly halts (see Figures 7-2A and 10-3). With increasing calcification and thickening, the valve cusps lose mobility and their excursion lessens; the click softens and ultimately may disappear.

An ejection sound is found less commonly in *acquired* aortic stenosis on a tricuspid aortic valve. The intensity of aortic closure (A_2) mirrors that of the aortic ejection sound. *Practical Point: Systolic clicks are present in less than one third of older patients with aortic stenosis (>50 years of age) but are the rule in congenital aortic stenosis.*

How to Listen to the Ejection Click or Sound

The ejection click is a high-frequency, crisp sound (see Figures 7-1 and 10-3). It occurs 40–80 msec after S_1, a longer interval than that separating the normal mitral and tricuspid components of S_1. Contrary to what one might expect, the aortic ejection sound usually is heard best *at the cardiac apex,* where it often is louder than both S_1 and S_2. A typical click has a "snappy" quality and is heard throughout the precordium. It is readily mistaken for S_1, particularly at the base of the heart.

Ejection sounds or clicks are not commonly considered or sought in routine cardiac auscultation. One should remember that a loudly "split" S_1 at the apex and lower left sternal border may represent an S_1 ejection click complex. The aortic ejection click does not vary with inspiration as opposed to the pulmonic ejection sound.

Murmur

Aortic stenosis produces the prototype of the classic systolic ejection murmur: a crescendo-decrescendo murmur that begins after S_1 and ends before S. The murmur typically is harsh, rough, or grunting and maximal at the second left interspace. It has been likened to the sound of someone clearing his or her throat. Although the classic aortic stenosis murmur is virtually diagnostic, a number of factors may alter the usual findings.

Site of Maximal Intensity

In most subjects, the murmur will be loudest at the second right interspace, the so-called aortic area. However, it is not uncommon for the murmur to be maximal at the second or third left interspace (Erb's point), and in older patients with large chests or obstructive lung disease, the murmur may be loudest at the apex. Therefore, it is best to think of distribution and radiation of the aortic stenosis murmur as a "sash pattern" that extends from the aortic area downward to the left and to the cardiac apex. The murmur at the cardiac base typically radiates upward and to the right and is heard well over both carotid arteries.

Length of Murmur

In general, the length of the murmur is proportional to the severity of the valvular obstruction in the absence of other factors that modify stroke volume or the rate of ejection (see Figure 10-5). The presence of associated aortic insufficiency usually produces a louder murmur due to the increased stroke volume. In the presence of decreased left ventricular function or overt congestive heart failure, the murmur of aortic stenosis may shorten or completely disappear.

The time to the peak intensity of the murmur may be a better indicator of severity of aortic stenosis than its overall length. *Practical Point: It is important to assess the duration to the maximal murmur intensity in the evaluation of the severity of aortic stenosis. A murmur that peaks within the first third or half of systole suggests mild obstruction. A murmur that peaks within the second half of systole indicates severe disease* (see Figure 10-5).

Murmur Frequency and Pitch

The typical rough, grunting quality of the murmur of aortic stenosis is heard best at the aortic area. It has long been observed that, in adults with acquired aortic stenosis, the systolic murmur at the apex can be quite musical in its pure frequency and high-pitched sound (the Gallavardin murmur). This is often so dramatic that the systolic murmurs at the aortic area and the apex are thought to be two separate murmurs, the latter typically confused with mitral regurgitation. It is thus important to recognize that in older patients, particularly those with an increased chest diameter, the systolic murmur of aortic stenosis may be markedly different in tone at the base and apex, although the shape and length of the murmur is similar (ejection).

Amplitude

In general, the louder is the murmur of aortic stenosis, the more severe the valve obstruction. This observation probably is more true in children or young adults with bicuspid valves in whom a loud murmur almost always indicates a large aortic gradient. This relationship is less reliable in adults, as evidenced by the soft or unimpressive murmur occasionally found in patients with severe aortic stenosis. In the presence of chronic obstructive lung disease, obesity, or a big chest it is important to auscultate at the base with the patient upright and leaning forward. The murmur of aortic stenosis in such individuals often is heard very well over and above the clavicles (bone is a good sound conductor) and in the neck. Conversely, in such patients or in the presence of congestive heart failure or those with coexisting mitral stenosis, the finding of a prominent grade 3–4 murmur of aortic stenosis is a most important observation that suggests severe aortic valvular obstruction. The systolic murmur usually is quite soft and unimpressive in these situations, giving the false impression that aortic stenosis is mild or absent.

Associated Aortic Regurgitation

Many patients, particularly those with rheumatic heart disease, have some degree of aortic regurgitation even in the presence of severe aortic stenosis. The rigid, contracted, and often calcified valve may be truly immobile, unable to adequately open or close (see Figure 10-1B). It is common for a trivial degree of aortic regurgitation to coexist with severe aortic stenosis (LV-aortic gradient greater than 75 mmHg), resulting in a grade 1–2/6 high-frequency aortic regurgitation blow. *Practical Point: While using firm pressure with the diaphragm of the stethoscope, specifically listen for a blowing diastolic murmur in all patients with suspected aortic stenosis by having the subject sit up and lean forward with the breath held in expiration.* The presence of aortic regurgitation of any magnitude will tend to augment the stroke volume and therefore the intensity and length of the systolic murmur for any degree of valve obstruction.

Differential Diagnosis

Aortic Sclerosis or the Systolic Murmur of the Elderly

The systolic murmur common in older persons results from the stiffening of the basal aspects of the aortic valve leaflets without commissural fusion; thickening of the leaflet tissue and even calcification can be present. There is no actual valve obstruction or aortic gradient. The murmur of aortic sclerosis is that of a classic systolic ejection murmur of less than grade 4/6 intensity. A_2 typically is well preserved. The carotids have a brisk upstroke. There is no evidence of left ventricular enlargement on precordial palpation. Most important, the overall length and peak intensity of the murmur fall within the first half of systole. Nevertheless, the differential diagnosis can be most difficult at times.

Mitral Regurgitation

When an aortic stenosis murmur radiates to the apex or is louder at the apex, the differential diagnosis should include mitral regurgitation. This is a particular problem in the older patient or the subject with a large chest, where the apical aortic murmur is likely to be of a higher frequency and have a more musical tone. To make the distinction between a murmur of aortic or mitral origin, it is critical to assess the length of the murmur and pay close attention to late systole. The murmur of aortic stenosis often is heard above the clavicles; the murmur of mitral regurgitation usually radiates well into the axilla. A normal carotid pulse favors mitral regurgitation.

If an arrhythmia is present, an accurate diagnosis may be made more easily. The intensity of the aortic stenosis murmur varies directly with the magnitude of the LV stroke volume, whereas a mitral regurgitation murmur tends to be equally loud as left ventricular volume changes on a beat-to-beat basis. Therefore, in a post-PVC beat or following a long R-R cycle in atrial fibrillation, the murmur of aortic stenosis will increase in loudness, but there will be no change in intensity of the mitral regurgitation murmur.

11

Hypertrophic Cardiomyopathy

Hypertrophic cardiomyopathy, also known in the United States as *idiopathic hypertrophic subaortic stenosis* (IHSS), is one of the most unusual cardiac disorders. Its precise etiology and pathophysiology remain to be fully elucidated.

The hallmark of hypertrophic cardiomyopathy (HC) is the presence of massive interventricular septal thickening, typically in the superior portion of the muscular septum (Figure 11-1). There usually is associated distortion of the mitral valve apparatus, resulting in an abnormally displaced anterolateral papillary muscle and anterior leaflet of the mitral valve. The anterior mitral cusp is distorted by vigorous left ventricular contraction and may be displaced toward the interventricular septum during systole; some believe that the mitral valve contributes to left ventricular blood flow "obstruction" during mid- to late ejection.

Hypertrophic cardiomyopathy has two major variants. The first variant is an *obstructive* form with a measurable pressure gradient at rest or with provocative maneuvers between the body of the left ventricle and the distal left ventricular outflow tract. The second variant is a *nonobstructive* form characterized by left ventricular hypertrophy, involving the interventricular septum as well as a portion of the left ventricular free wall, no resting or provokable intraventricular gradient, and relatively little abnormality of mitral valve structure or function.

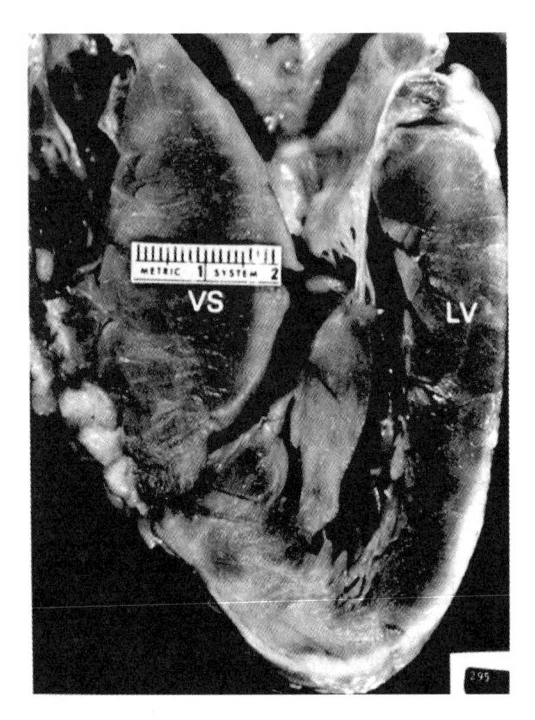

Figure 11-1. Massive ventricular septal thickening in hypertrophic cardiomyopathy. The septum bulges into the left ventricular cavity. The left ventricular free wall (LV) is hypertrophied and has a small left ventricular cavity. Asymmetric septal hypertrophy (VS) is prominent in most but not all cases. (Reprinted with permission from Maron BJ. Cardiomyopathies. In: Adams FH, Emmanouilides GC, eds. *Moss' Heart Disease in Infants, Children and Adolescents*, 3rd ed. Baltimore: Williams & Wilkins; 1983.)

Both the obstructive and nonobstructive variants of HC demonstrate hyperdynamic ejection characteristics with extremely rapid and forceful left ventricular contraction, especially in early systole.

Pathology

The typical heart in obstructive HC has dramatic asymmetric hypertrophy of the interventricular septum, with normal or somewhat hypertrophied left ventricular free walls (see Figure 11-1). The septal cardiac muscle is composed of striking myofiber disarray with loss of normal cellular architecture. Increased connective tissue is present. In patients with a measurable pressure gradient across the left ventricular outflow tract, the peculiar cellular pattern is confined to the massively hypertrophied septum, with normal cardiac muscle in the left ventricular free wall. The anterior leaflet of the mitral valve typically is thickened in HC, and the aortic valve is normal.

Pathophysiology

The dynamics of LV ejection in symptomatic patients with HC are similar and unrelated to the presence or absence of a left ventricular-aortic pressure gradient. Ejection of blood is extremely rapid and forceful, resulting in premature cavity emptying and an abnormally small LV end-systolic cavity. The left ventricle ejects 85–90% of its end-diastolic contents by the middle of systole. Ejection is virtually complete by two thirds of left ventricular systole. Normal persons, by contrast, eject 60% of the LV end-diastolic volume during the first half of systole and do not effectively complete emptying until 85–90% of systole has been completed.

Subjects with a large left ventricular-aortic pressure difference at rest or with provocation have the most prominent physical findings and almost always are symptomatic.

Anterior Leaflet of the Mitral Valve

A peculiar *systolic anterior motion* (SAM) is identified readily on echocardiography and angiography in obstructive HC. The anterior leaflet may make contact with the interventricular septum during mid- to late systole. SAM is found most commonly in patients with HC who have significant "obstruction" to outflow but may also be found in occasional patients with nonobstructive HC and *even those with mitral valve prolapse.*

Left Ventricular Compliance in Hypertrophic Cardiomyopathy

Some experts suggest that the predominant clinical effects of HC are not related to left ventricular outflow tract obstruction but are due to the profound alteration in compliance characteristics of the left ventricle in both the obstructive and nonobstructive variants. Thus, the extremely stiff, massively hypertrophied LV muscle resists diastolic inflow from the left atrium. Left ventricular filling pressure is abnormally high, with resultant elevation of pulmonary capillary pressure and enlargement of the left atrium.

Mitral Regurgitation

Mitral regurgitation occurs in 30–50% of affected subjects. Mitral regurgitation typically is found only in patients with a resting or provokable gradient, and its presence correlates with echocardiographic SAM.

Influences on the Pressure Gradient

A variety of agents and maneuvers affect the hemodynamics in hypertrophic cardiomyopathy (Table 11-1). Criley has used the term *ventriculovalvular disproportion* to emphasize that the left ventricular cavity actually is too small for the mitral valve in subjects with HC. Any maneuver or pharmacologic intervention that reduces left ventricular dimensions tends to increase or bring out a pressure gradient. The converse also is true. Increasing afterload or increasing end diastolic volume (preload) reduces the LV-aortic gradient. An agent or maneuver that augments cardiac contractility will increase the outflow gradient and accentuate the systolic murmur and other physical signs of HC.

Clinical Presentation

Hypertrophic cardiomyopathy represents a cardiac syndrome with a markedly variable course. Unique aspects of this condition are its unpredictability and the lack of an obvious correlation between the clinical manifestations of HC and the underlying hemodynamic profile as assessed by echocardiography or cardiac catheterization. Patients may die suddenly without having had any prior symptoms; there is no apparent relationship between these tragic sudden deaths and the presence or absence of obstruction in HC.

Table 11-1. Effects of Physiologic and Pharmacologic Maneuvers in Hypertrophic Cardiomyopathy

Intervention	Left Ventricular Outflow Obstruction	Murmur
Valsalva		
Strain	Increase	Increase (may also decrease)
Release	Decrease	Decrease
Squatting	Decrease	Decrease
Upright posture	Increase	Increase
Exercise	Increase	Increase
Amyl nitrite or nitroglycerin	Increase	Increase
Post-PVC	Increase	Increase

(Modified with permission from Shah PM. Newer concepts in hypertrophic obstructive cardiomyopathy. *JAMA.* 1979;242:1773.)

In asymptomatic individuals, HC usually is detected by accident, such as noting prominent precordial LV activity, an S_4, a loud systolic murmur, or an abnormal EKG. Some cases are recognized through screening of affected family members. Hypertrophic cardiomyopathy has been documented in the elderly. The diagnosis is easy to miss in a patient in the seventh or eighth decade of life because of a similarity of the clinical presentation to that of coronary or hypertensive heart disease (e.g., prominent LV, S_4, systolic murmur).

Presenting symptoms of HC include dyspnea on exertion, dizziness, syncope, angina, or palpitations. Shortness of breath is the most common symptom, a result of high LV filling pressures at rest or exercise due to the noncompliant, hypertrophied LV chamber. Dizziness and syncope may result from severe LV outflow tract obstruction or may be caused by arrhythmias. Angina may occur as a result of the increased myocardial oxygen demands of the hypertrophied ventricle with no commensurate increase in coronary blood flow. Sudden death, often occurring in young adults, usually is caused by malignant ventricular dysrhythmia.

Physical Examination

Jugular Venous Pulse

A large A wave is common as a result of noncompliant RV myocardium and powerful right atrial contraction. The mean jugular venous pressure is normal.

Carotid Arterial Pulse

The typical carotid pulse in HC reflects the early, exaggerated systolic emptying of the LV. It has a brisk or sharp upstroke that actually taps against the palpating fingers. *Practical Point: The presence of a brisk carotid arterial pulse contour in a patient being evaluated for possible aortic valve stenosis immediately should raise the suspicion of hypertrophic cardiomyopathy, particularly if there is a prominent systolic murmur.*

A bifid carotid arterial pulse often is recorded in HC, particularly in the obstructive variety. This is not easily appreciated on examination. The classic pulse contour consists of a rapid upstroke, followed by a midsystolic dip or collapse, which in turn is followed by a second, late-systolic wave (Figure 11-2).

Practical Point: The cardinal arterial pulse alteration in hypertrophic cardiomyopathy is a rapid, jerky, or sharp carotid pulse. The arterial pulse wave contour often is normal to palpation, especially in the absence of a resting gradient.

A thrill or shudder rarely is felt over the carotid arteries in nonobstructive or obstructive HC, in contradistinction to valvular aortic stenosis.

Precordial Motion

Abnormal precordial LV activity is common in subjects with HC, and this may be an important first clue that something is not quite right in the evaluation of a young patient with a systolic ejection murmur. The hallmark of precordial examination is the ubiquitous presence of a loud and typically palpable S_4 (presystolic distention of the LV) accompanied by a late-systolic apical heave, thrust, or bulge (Figure 11-3).

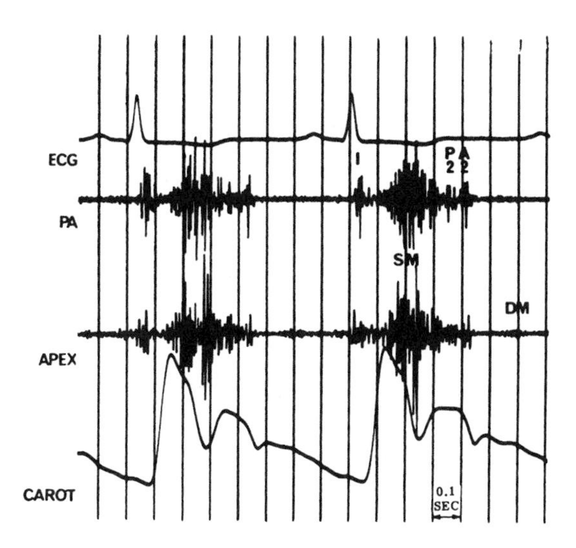

Figure 11-2. Apical impulse in hypertrophic cadiomyopathy. Note the large A wave or palpable S_4 and the prominent late systolic bulge. The systolic murmur is long and late peaking, suggesting significant obstruction to left ventricular outflow. (Reprinted with permission from Delman AJ, Stein E. *Dynamic Cardiac Auscultation and Phonocardiography*. Philadelphia: WB Saunders Co.; 1979.)

There may be an early systolic dip or retraction of the apical impulse, followed by an anterior midsystolic bulge or thrust. The combined presence of a palpable S_4 (normal), early-systolic impulse, and a late-systolic bulge may produce a trifid contour to the apex impulse; this has been called the *triple ripple*.

The typical LV impulse in HC is sustained, forceful, and palpable in more than one interspace. It is particularly prominent in the left decubitus position. A systolic thrill often is palpable and directly related to the presence and severity of a resting gradient. The thrill may be maximal at the lower left sternal border or at the apex. It is rarely felt at the base, in contrast to valvular aortic stenosis. *Practical Point: The presence of a systolic thrill in hypertrophic cardiomyopathy suggests that the patient has obstruction to left ventricular outflow.*

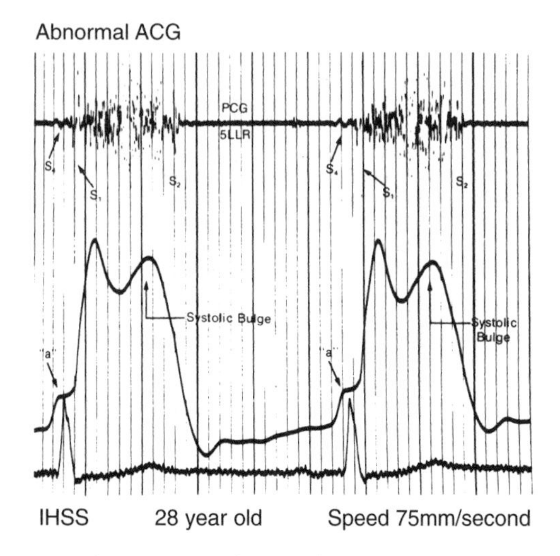

Figure 11-3. Typical murmur and arterial pulse in hypertrophic cardiomyopathy. Note the systolic ejection murmur that begins after S_1 and ends just before A_2. The carotid pulse shows the characteristic "spike and dome" configuration. S_2 demonstrates paradoxic splitting following a long, late-peaking murmur. These findings suggest significant "obstruction" to left ventricular outflow. (Reprinted with permission from Tavel ME. Phonocardiography: Clinical use with and without combined echocardiography. *Prog Cardiovasc Dis.* 1983;26:145.)

Heart Sounds

First Heart Sound

The first heart sound is normal or accentuated in HC.

Second Heart Sound

Left ventricular ejection usually is prolonged and, as a result, S_2 often is narrowly split with inspiration. When significant obstruction is present, A_2 may be delayed beyond P_2 and reversed or paradoxic splitting of S_2 appears. *Practical Point: Usually there is no diagnostic abnormality of the second heart sound in hypertrophic cardiomyopathy. Reversed splitting of S_2, when present, suggests a large left ventricular-aortic gradient.*

Third Heart Sound

An S_3 in HC occasionally is noted. When present, the S_3 does not indicate poor left ventricular function but may reflect the profound alteration in left ventricular diastolic compliance. An S_3 is more likely when there is associated mitral regurgitation. In one large study, an S_3 was recorded in over half the patients with HC, most of whom had a resting pressure gradient.

Fourth Heart Sound

An S_4 commonly is heard or palpated in obstructive or nonobstructive HC (see Figure 11-3). The presence of a prominent atrial sound in a young subject with a systolic murmur should initiate a careful examination for HC. A loud S_4 is related to augmented left atrial contraction and the typically stiff and hypertrophied LV. *Practical Point: Be wary of making the diagnosis of hypertrophic cardiomyopathy in any person who has no S_4. A loud atrial sound is the rule in this disorder.*

The Systolic Murmur

The characteristic murmur of obstructive hypertrophic cardiomyopathy is a long, somewhat harsh systolic ejection murmur (see Figures 11-2 and 11-3). It is well heard at the apex and lower left sternal border and may be extremely variable in intensity. In patients with a large pressure gradient across the left ventricular outflow tract, the murmur tends to peak in late systole. In mild degrees of outflow tract obstruction, a soft, late-peaking systolic murmur may be heard. In general, with increasing severity of the gradient the murmur becomes louder and longer.

Timing

The murmur of HC typically has a crescendo-decrescendo shape, peaking late in systole in the obstructive variant and ending before A_2 (see Figures 11-2 and 11-3). When there is associated mitral regurgitation, the murmur may seem longer at the apex than at the base.

On auscultation, such murmurs appear to be holosystolic, often with a tapering configuration in late systole. It is unusual to hear the classic whirring pansystolic murmur of mitral regurgitation in HC. In addition, the systolic murmur of HC typically begins *after* S_1, even in subjects with documented mitral incompetence. The physician should focus intently on early and late systole to assess the duration of the murmur.

In patients with no obstruction or those with a small gradient, the systolic murmur is shorter and even may be absent. Asymptomatic subjects with echo-proven asymmetrical septal hypertrophy but no other evidence of HC often have no murmur suggestive of this disorder.

Intensity

The amplitude of the HC murmur is extremely variable. It may change as much as one or two grades with a change in body position or exaggerated respiration. The murmur may vary in intensity and length from day to day or even hour to hour. Various maneuvers or agents may be utilized to augment the loudness of the murmur in patients suspected of having HC (see the section on physical maneuvers and pharmacologic agents, see Table 11-1).

Loud murmurs typically are associated with a measurable outflow gradient and may have an accompanying systolic thrill. A thrill suggests a large gradient.

Location and Radiation

The systolic murmur in HC is best heard in the lower, midprecordial area between the apex and lower left sternal border. Usually, it is maximal close to the sternum in the third to fourth left interspace at a site considerably lower than the location of the typical murmur of valvular aortic stenosis. Less commonly, the murmur is loudest at or just inside the apex. The murmur usually does not radiate well to the aortic area and neck and rarely is prominent over the carotid arteries or in the suprasternal area.

When mitral regurgitation is associated with obstructive HC, the systolic murmur often appears to be longer and may be heard best at the cardiac apex. It may radiate into the axilla. *Practical Point: Hypertrophic cardiomyopathy should be considered whenever a systolic murmur appears to have both ejection and regurgitant characteristics with the site of maximal intensity lower than the site of a typical ejection murmur.*

Physical Maneuvers and Pharmacologic Agents Used in Diagnosis

Transient hemodynamic alterations produced by altered physiology can produce striking changes in the physical findings in hypertrophic cardiomyopathy (see Table 11-1 and Figure 11-4). The use of various maneuvers and drugs has been most informative in our understanding of the basic pathophysiology of this fascinating condition. Any intervention

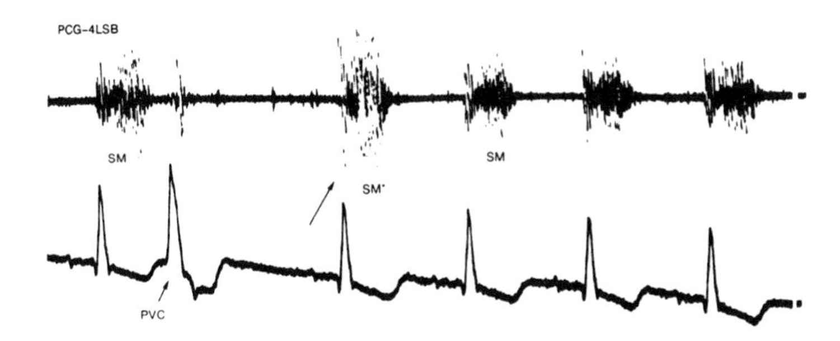

Figure 11-4. Post-PVC augmentation of the systolic murmur (SM) in hypertrophic cardiomyopathy. Note the accentuation of the murmur that occurs in the beat following the PVC. Augmentation of the murmur is related to increased "obstruction" to left ventricular outflow in the post-PVC beat. (Reprinted with permission from Delman AJ, Stein E. *Dynamic Cardiac Auscultation and Phonocardiography*. Philadelphia: WB Saunders Co.; 1979.)

that increases the resting outflow tract gradient in a patient with "obstructive" HC or that can initiate a pressure gradient when there is no resting gradient will accentuate or produce the systolic murmur. The murmur typically will become louder and longer and peak later in systole (see Figure 11-4). The converse is also true: Maneuvers that decrease the left ventricular outflow tract gradient will reduce the amplitude and length of the systolic murmur and minimize other features of the cardiac examination associated with obstruction. On occasion, however, provocation of a markedly increased gradient (Valsalva maneuver, post-PVC beat) will result in no change or even a decrease in the murmur.

One can predict what will happen to the pressure gradient and the quality of the murmur in a patient suspected or known to have obstructive hypertrophic cardiomyopathy by remembering the following guidelines.

The magnitude of the gradient and the systolic murmur are accentuated by anything that causes

1. A reduction in left ventricular cavity volume or pressure (decreased preload).
2. A decrease in systemic vascular resistance or arterial pressure (decreased afterload).
3. An increase in the left ventricular contractile state.

Conversely, apparent obstruction to left ventricular outflow is reduced and the systolic murmur softens as a result of

1. An increase in left ventricular cavity volume or filling pressure.
2. An increase in systemic arterial pressure or resistance.
3. A drug or intervention that decreases left ventricular contractility.

A smaller left ventricular outflow tract and small left ventricular cavity in systole accentuates the ventricular-valvular disproportion and exaggerates the pressure gradient, whether present or latent. Such murmur variations are similar to the behavior of the systolic murmur of mitral valve prolapse.

Changes in the distending forces exerted on the distal left ventricular outflow tract and central aorta beyond the site of intracavitary obstruction alters the gradient across the left ventricular outflow tract. An increase in aortic pressure "opens up" the distal outflow tract, helps push the anterior leaflet of the mitral valve posteriorly toward the left atrium, and reduces any existing or latent obstruction. Conversely, a decrease in aortic pressure or vascular resistance enhances anterior displacement of the mitral leaflet toward the septum and increases the gradient.

The maneuvers and pharmacologic agents listed in Table 11-1 are particularly helpful when a diagnosis of hypertrophic cardiomyopathy is being considered. Use of these interventions often clarifies the clinical situation; the diagnosis of HC may be influenced by behavior of the murmur with various interventions.

The use of the Valsalva maneuver is recommended for optimal diagnostic utility. An equivocal or soft murmur of HC should become much louder.

Differential Diagnosis

The systolic murmur of HC commonly is confused with valvular aortic stenosis, mitral regurgitation, or a ventricular septal defect. Careful synthesis of all the physical findings usually can differentiate these entities, although echocardiography may be required as the final arbiter. The sequelae of coronary artery disease occasionally can be confused with HC.

Valvular Aortic Stenosis

The cardinal differential feature between HC and aortic stenosis is the quality of the carotid pulse. In obstructive HC, the carotid upstroke is quick and the pulse volume normal. In aortic stenosis, the upstroke is delayed, often slurred, and the pulse volume is reduced (see Figure 10-3). The murmur of aortic valve stenosis usually is heard well at the base and radiates into the neck; in HC, the murmur optimally is detected lower in the precordium and, as a rule, radiates poorly to the base. Post-PVC augmentation typically is more prominent in HC than in valvular stenosis (see Figure 11-4). The classic response to Valsalva strain is opposite in the two conditions (at least 20–30% of HC patients show no increase in murmur intensity with Valsalva). The presence of a high-frequency aortic ejection click or the murmur of aortic regurgitation is good evidence against HC as the primary diagnosis.

Mitral Regurgitation

Chronic mitral regurgitation may simulate HC. A holosystolic murmur at the apex indicates the presence of mitral regurgitation, with or without a left ventricular outflow tract gradient. An audible or palpable S_4 is distinctly unusual in chronic mitral regurgitation but common in acute onset mitral reflux (see Chapter 13). Evidence for left ventricular hypertrophy usually is much more prominent in HC than in chronic mitral regurgitation. The quality of the carotid pulse may be similar in both conditions but usually has a quicker rise in HC. Reversed splitting of S_2 is not a feature of mitral regurgitation. The response to amyl nitrite, Valsalva maneuver, and the post-PVC beat should be useful in the differential diagnosis; the murmur of pure mitral regurgitation behaves in a direction opposite to the responses in HC (see Table 11-1). Squatting decreases the HC murmur and increases that of mitral regurgitation; standing results in directionally opposite changes.

Mitral Valve Prolapse

The murmur of mitral valve prolapse behaves similarly to HC in many maneuvers (Valsalva, standing, squatting), but the absence of prominent

LV hypertrophy and an S_4 and the presence of a midsystolic click easily should differentiate the late-systolic murmur of mitral prolapse from HC.

Hypertensive Heart Disease

In older patients with long-standing hypertension and a prominent left ventricular impulse, an ejection murmur and the presence of an S_4 may suggest hypertrophic cardiomyopathy. This can be a difficult diagnostic dilemma. Attention to the carotid pulse contour and response to maneuvers and amyl nitrite will aid in the differential diagnosis.

12

Aortic Regurgitation

Aortic regurgitation (AR) is associated with a variety of underlying disorders. Acute aortic regurgitation can be life threatening. The physical findings in severe chronic aortic regurgitation are striking and have fascinated physicians for centuries.

Etiology

Rheumatic heart disease remains the most common cause of aortic regurgitation, but many other conditions can produce an incompetent aortic valve such as endocarditis, syphilis, cystic medial necrosis of the aorta, congenital deformities (bicuspid aortic valve is the most common), and diseases of the aortic root. The last category includes aneurysms of the aorta or sinus of Valsalva but usually is idiopathic. Acute aortic regurgitation can be produced by blunt or penetrating trauma, endocarditis, or dissection.

Pathophysiology

Aortic regurgitation results from failure of the aortic valve leaflets to remain competent during diastole, allowing reflux of blood into the left ventricle. The regurgitation may be caused by a tear or perforation of a single aortic valve cusp or may result from a more diffuse process that affects the valve leaflets, the aortic ring, or both. Intrinsic disease of the aortic root (e.g., aneurysm, dissection) can produce aortic regurgitation in the presence of normal valve leaflets when the proximal aorta is sufficiently dilated or distorted.

The severity of aortic regurgitation is directly related to the amount of ejected stroke volume that refluxes back into the left ventricle during diastole. In severe or "free" aortic regurgitation, well over half of the ejected stroke volume refluxes back into the left ventricle.

Aortic regurgitation produces a classic *volume overload* state. The left ventricle initially dilates and ejects more blood per beat: Stroke volume remains proportional to the regurgitant volume until left ventricular decompensation occurs. Eccentric left ventricular hypertrophy results, with prominent chamber enlargement and a proportionately smaller increase in wall thickness. There is an increase in left ventricular compliance in chronic aortic regurgitation; left ventricular filling pressure remains relatively normal in the presence of considerable ventricular dilatation. Cardiac output is maintained, and the ejection rate and ejection fraction actually is increased in early or mild aortic regurgitation. In time, however, major aortic incompetence results in a decrease in the compliance of the ventricle with subsequent elevation of left ventricular filling pressure. At this point, patients typically become symptomatic; congestive heart failure may result when left ventricular contractility becomes sufficiently impaired.

Acute Aortic Regurgitation

In acute aortic incompetence, the physical findings may be substantially different from those of chronic regurgitation (discussed later in this chapter). When the left ventricle is challenged abruptly with a severe diastolic overload, normal compensatory mechanisms lack the time to develop. The LV is unable to adequately handle the large regurgitant flow, and the left ventricular filling pressure becomes markedly elevated. The effective cardiac output falls. Peripheral vascular signs of severe aortic regurgitation are attenuated or may never appear due to marked systemic vasoconstriction. The heart rate usually is increased. Left ventricular failure in this clinical context carries a grave prognosis. Therefore, early recognition of acute aortic regurgitation is imperative.

Physical Examination

Blood Pressure

The systemic blood pressure is a valuable clue to the degree of aortic regurgitation. With progressive severity of aortic reflux, the systolic blood pressure increases and the aortic diastolic pressure declines (Figure 12-1). *Practical Point: The presence of a completely normal blood pressure in a patient with aortic regurgitation and excellent left ventricular function virtually excludes moderate to severe aortic incompetence.* In hemodynamically significant aortic regurgitation, diastolic pressure typically falls below 70 mmHg and systolic pressure may rise to 140–150 mmHg. Systolic pressure will not increase more than 150–160 mmHg in the absence of associated systemic hypertension.

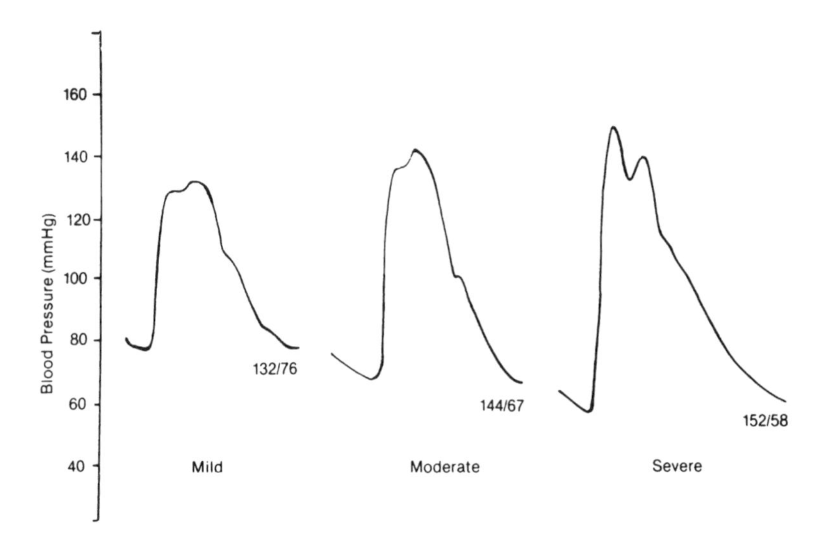

Figure 12-1. The arterial pulse and blood pressure in aortic regurgitation. There is little alteration in the arterial pulse and pressure in mild aortic regurgitation. With increasing reflux across the aortic valve, systolic blood pressure increases and diastolic blood pressure decreases, resulting in widening of the pulse pressure. The increased left ventricular stroke volume results in high-amplitude, palpable arterial pulsation with rapid falloff in late systole. This adds a collapsing quality to the pulse. In severe aortic regurgitation, arterial pulsations are prominent and often visible in the peripheral circulation as well.

The degree of decrease in diastolic blood pressure is a better benchmark for assessing the severity of aortic regurgitation than the increase in systolic pressure. In severe or "free" aortic incompetence, the diastolic blood pressure ranges from 40 to 50 mmHg, approaching or equaling the markedly elevated LVEDP. It is best to use the point of *muffling* of Korotkoff sounds as the indication of diastolic blood pressure in subjects with aortic regurgitation; audible sounds may be detected to zero.

Practical Point: Severe isolated aortic regurgitation uncommonly will be present in a patient with a diastolic blood pressure greater than 60 mmHg if there is no evidence of reduced left ventricular pump function or systemic hypertension. Conversely, a diastolic blood pressure of 50 mmHg or less almost always indicates a major degree of aortic incompetence, irrespective of the level of systolic pressure.

Carotid Arterial Pulse

The large stroke volume and enhanced rate of ejection produced by hemodynamically significant aortic regurgitation results in a characteristic *high-amplitude arterial pulse* (see Figure 12-1). The pulse has a *collapsing* quality caused by the low systemic vascular resistance and early diastolic reflux of blood into the left ventricle, which result in rapid "unloading" into the aorta. With a very large stroke volume, the pulse is full, actually swelling under the examining finger, then rapidly abating. Pulsation of proximal carotid arteries may be visible (Corrigan's sign). Patients may be conscious of this arterial throbbing. Arterial pulses throughout the body are increased in force and amplitude and display a typical bounding quality.

Bisferiens Pulse

One of the hallmarks of aortic regurgitation is the bisferiens, or double systolic, arterial pulse (Figure 12-2). This bifid pulsation is best felt with light finger pressure over the carotid arteries. On occasion, a transmitted systolic thrill or bruit also is felt, making precise identification of the bisferiens contour difficult. In severe aortic regurgitation, a systolic shudder of the carotid artery may be noted with or without associated aortic stenosis. The bisferiens pulse is present only in moderate to severe aortic regurgitation or in patients with aortic regurgitation and associated mild aortic stenosis.

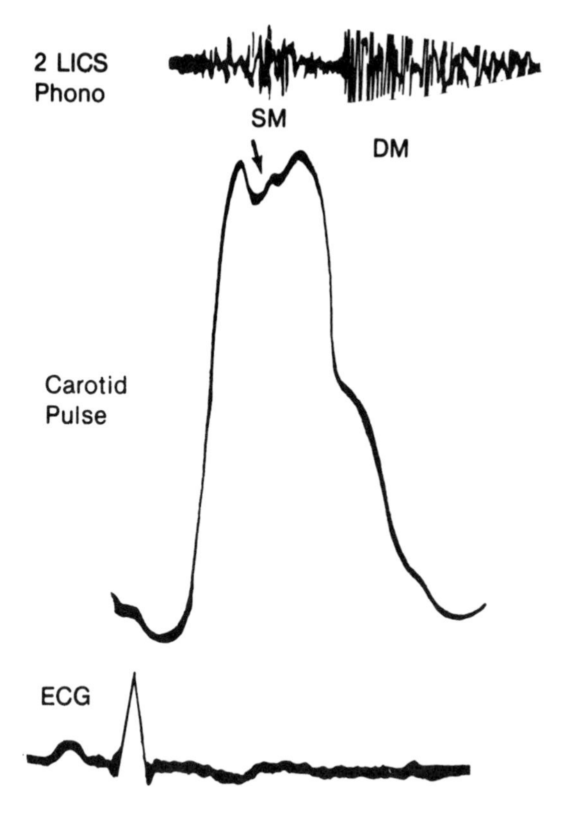

Figure 12-2. Bisferiens pulse of aortic regurgitation. Note the bifid systolic pulse wave, which is detected best using light finger pressure over the carotid arteries. This contour is associated with increased pulse volume. The bisferiens pulse must be differentiated from a transmitted systolic murmur or palpable thrill. Note the soft S_1 and S_2. SM = systolic murmur; DM = diastolic murmur; 2 LICS = second left intercostal space.

Peripheral Signs

Major degrees of aortic incompetence produce a variety of abnormalities directly related to forceful ejection of an increased stroke volume into a dilated arterial bed. The abrupt rise and fall of the arterial pulse wave causes a distinctive pounding or collapsing quality that is accentuated in the peripheral arteries. Marked systemic vasodilation may produce noncardiac phenomena, such as increased sweating, warm flushed skin, and accentuated retinal vein pulsations.

Many well-known eponyms have been given to these *nonauscultatory signs of aortic regurgitation.* In general, the presence of such peripheral abnormalities correlates well with the increased systolic and pulse pressure and decreased diastolic pressure common to advanced aortic regurgitation. *Practical Point: Nonauscultatory signs are never seen in mild aortic regurgitation but are the rule in chronic severe aortic incompetence in the absence of congestive heart failure.* Low cardiac output or the onset of heart failure may attenuate these signs. Table 12-1 lists most of the peripheral abnormalities that have been described in aortic regurgitation and their eponyms.

Table 12-1. Peripheral or Nonauscultatory Signs of Severe Aortic Regurgitation: A Glossary of Terms

Bisferiens pulse	A double or bifid systolic impulse felt in the arterial pulse.
Corrigan's sign	Visible pulsations of the supraclavicular and carotid arteries.
Pistol shot of Traube	A loud systolic sound heard with the stethoscope lightly placed over the femoral arteries.
Palmar click	A palpable, abrupt flushing of the palms in systole.
Quincke's pulse	Exaggerated sequential reddening and blanching of the fingernail beds when light pressure is applied to the tip of the fingernail. A similar observation can be made by pressing a glass slide to the lips.
Duroziez's sign	A to-and-fro bruit heard over the femoral artery when light pressure is applied to the artery by the edge of the stethoscope head. The bruit is caused by the exaggerated reversal of flow in diastole.
de Musset's sign	Visible oscillation or bobbing of the head with each heart beat.
Hill's sign	Abnormal accentuation of leg systolic blood pressure, with popliteal pressure 40 mmHg or higher than brachial artery pressure.
Water-hammer pulse	The high amplitude, abruptly collapsing pulse of aortic regurgitation. The term refers to a popular Victorian toy comprising a glass vessel partially filled with water that produced a slapping impact on being turned over.
Müller's sign	Visible pulsations of the uvula.

Precordial Motion

The quality of the left ventricular impulse parallels the severity of the aortic regurgitation. In mild to moderate aortic regurgitation, the left ventricular impulse is normal in size (Figure 12-3A) but often hyperdynamic. Therefore, the amplitude is exaggerated, but there is no leftward displacement of the apex beat; the apical impulse falls away from the palpating finger by midsystole (Figure 12-3B). With greater degrees of aortic regurgitation, the hyperkinetic impulse becomes more prominent, and the cardiac apex is displaced inferolaterally. When LV dilatation or a decrease in the ejection fraction occurs, typically with an increased end-systolic volume, the apex beat becomes *sustained* (Figure 12-3C). In patients with very large hearts or significant depression of left ventricular function, a prolonged and forceful LV lift or heave is predictable, and this finding may be impressive.

In severe aortic regurgitation, the apex impulse typically is found in the left anterior axillary line at the fifth or sixth interspace, usually occupies at least two interspaces, and is sustained into late systole. Not uncommonly, a palpable S_4 (presystolic distention) may be noted in the left decubitus position (see Figures 12-3C and 6-2). A visible and palpable rapid LV filling wave (S_3) may be detected in severe aortic regurgitation.

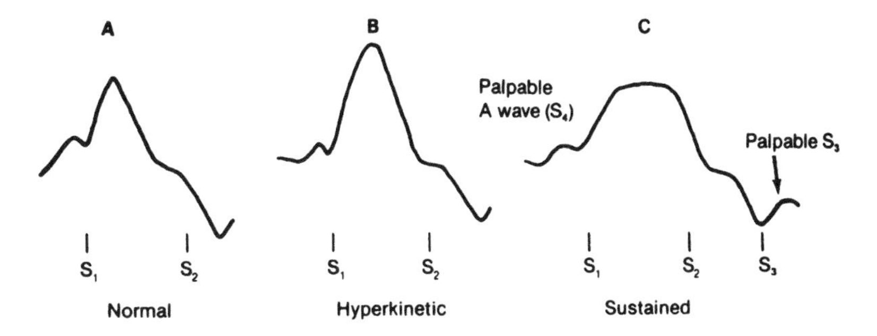

Figure 12-3. Precordial motion patterns in aortic regurgitation. (A) In mild regurgitation, the left ventricular impulse is normal. (B) As the left ventricle dilates with increasing volume overload, the apical impulse becomes more forceful with a higher amplitude (hyperkinetic impulse). Outward precordial motion still is felt only in early systole. The site of the PMI may be displaced laterally and downward. (C) A sustained left ventricular impulse will be felt when the ventricular cavity is substantially enlarged. At this stage, left ventricular contactility and ejection fraction may be preserved or abnormally depressed. The PMI always is displaced to the left and inferiorly at this state, and the force of the apical impulse is usually increased.

Heart Sounds

First Heart Sound

S_1 has a normal intensity in mild to moderate cases but often is decreased in severe aortic regurgitation (Figure 12-4). An aortic ejection sound easily is mistaken for S_1 in aortic regurgitation; this can give a false impression of a normal or even loud S_1. Whenever "S_1" is particularly prominent at the base in patients with aortic incompetence; it is likely due to an aortic ejection click instead of S_1.

Second Heart Sound

The aortic component of S_2 is variable in intensity in patients with aortic regurgitation. Although many textbooks have emphasized an increased amplitude of A_2, recent work indicates the A_2 may be *softer* than usual in aortic regurgitation because of a decreased ability of the valve leaflets to vibrate after aortic valve closure. In patients with moderate to severe aortic regurgitation, S_2 often is single.

Third Heart Sound

An S_3 is not a feature of mild to moderate aortic incompetence. However, in severe aortic regurgitation, an S_3 is common (see Figure 12-4). The increase in LV diastolic blood volume in part is responsible for the prominent S_3; left ventricular dilatation and decreased contractility may be significant additive factors. The S_3 frequently is a visible and palpable event, coinciding with the rapid filling phase of left ventricular diastole. An S_3 is more likely to be heard in younger patients. An S_3 is an adverse prognostic marker in severe aortic regurgitation.

Fourth Heart Sound

While an atrial sound is an uncommon finding in mild aortic regurgitation, it may be found occasionally in moderate aortic incompetence and is common in severe disease. The long PR interval common in many patients with aortic regurgitation increases audibility of an S_4. The S_4 may be manifest at the apex as palpable presystolic distention when the patient is turned onto his or her left side (see Figures 6-2 and 12-3C).

Aortic Ejection Click

An aortic ejection click or sound is detectable in many subjects with aortic regurgitation. More commonly it is heard in mild disease when there is good left ventricular function. The ejection click may be of

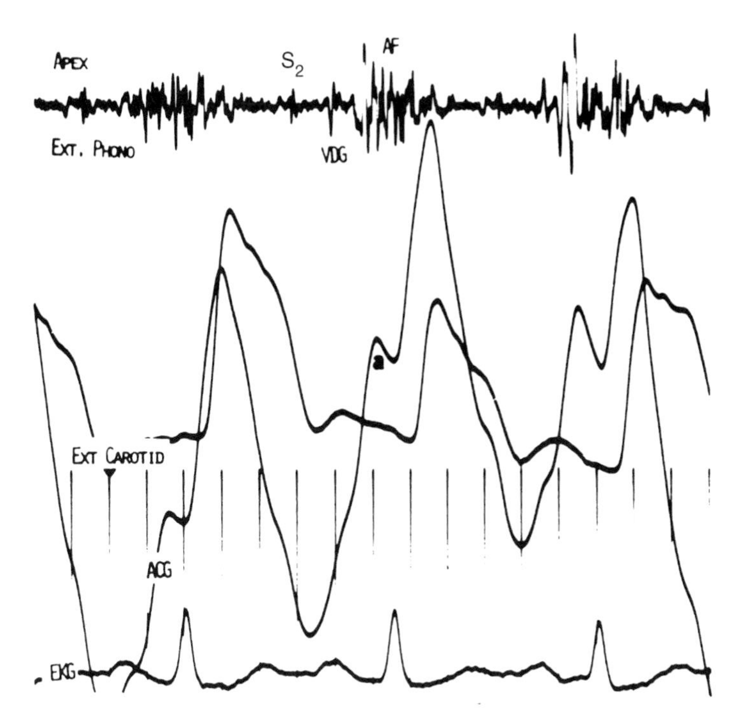

Figure 12-4. Third heart sound and Austin Flint murmur in acute aortic regurgitation. This phonocardiogram demonstrates an S_3 or ventricular diastolic gallop (VDG) followed by a loud Austin Flint murmur (AF) extending into late diastole. Note the accentuation of this murmur with atrial systole. The apex cardiogram (ACG) reveals a markedly augmented A wave and hyperdynamic LV impulse. S_1 is virtually absent. The auscultatory findings in such a patient may be extremely difficult to interpret. The presence of an S_3 and an Austin Flint murmur in acute or chronic aortic regurgitation indicates a major degree of aortic reflux. (Reprinted with permission from Reddy PS et al. Syndrome of acute aortic regurgitation. In: Leon DF, Shaver JA, eds. *Physiologic Principles of Heart Sounds and Murmurs.* American Heart Association Monograph No. 46. Armonk, NY: Futura; 1975.)

valve or root origin. When there is a bicuspid valve, the ejection click is produced by the maximal opening excursion of the abnormal valve cusps. In subjects with an enlarged, abnormal aortic root, the ejection sound most likely is produced by sudden systolic expansion of the ascending aorta itself during early ejection (see Figure 7-2B). A snappy or prominently split S_1 or an S_1 that is heard well at the base in a patient with aortic regurgitation should suggest to the clinician that the S_1 actually is an aortic ejection click.

Cardiac Murmurs

Three different murmurs may be found in patients with aortic regurgitation: (1) the classic decrescendo diastolic murmur resulting from reflux of blood into the left ventricle; (2) a systolic ejection murmur produced by the large stroke volume, increased rate of ejection, and abnormal valve anatomy; (3) the Austin Flint murmur, a low-pitched diastolic murmur beginning in middiastole and found only in major degrees of aortic regurgitation.

Diastolic Murmur

The typical diastolic murmur of aortic regurgitation has a decrescendo shape (see Figures 12-2 and 12-5). The volume and velocity of refluxing blood across the incompetent aortic valve tapers off in mid- to late diastole as the aortic-left ventricular pressure gradient decreases. *In general, the length of the AR murmur is dependent on the severity of the leak except in very severe aortic regurgitation* (see later and Figure 12-5). The classic finding in AR is a diastolic murmur that tapers during diastole and may or may not extend to S_1.

Frequency

The diastolic murmur typically is high frequency or "blowing" in quality in mild to moderate aortic regurgitation. It is important to auscultate as the patient holds his or her breath in held expiration so as not to confuse the AR murmur with the noise of breathing. *Practical Point: The high-frequency murmur of mild aortic regurgitation frequently is soft. As most physicians are unaccustomed to hearing sounds of such high pitch, this faint AR murmur easily is missed by the unsuspecting examiner.* Echocardiographic studies have confirmed that minimal to mild aortic regurgitation is frequently silent. With more severe degrees of AR, low to medium frequency sound vibrations occur, and the murmur may be surprisingly low pitched.

Duration

In mild degrees of aortic regurgitation (regurgitant fraction of less than 0.3–0.4), the diastolic murmur may not be audible in late diastole, although a large gradient between the aorta and left ventricle persists throughout diastole (Figure 12-5A). In fact, the murmur of

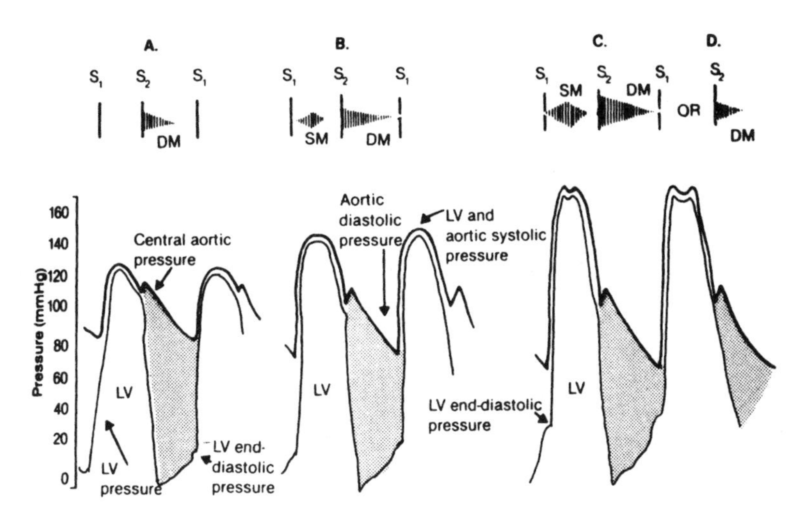

Figure 12-5. Diastolic and systolic murmurs of aortic regurgitation. This diagram shows the relationship between the severity of aortic regurgitation, hemodynamic findings, and the characteristic murmurs of mild, moderate, and severe aortic regurgitation. (A) Mild aortic regurgitation: The diastolic gradient between the aorta and left ventricle is large; reflux of blood is high in velocity and small in volume. The resultant diastolic murmur (DM) is of variable length and high frequency. A systolic ejection murmur (SM) may not be present. (B) Moderate aortic insufficiency: The diastolic murmur is decrescendo and invariably long. The murmur may have medium- or high-frequency vibrations. A systolic ejection (flow) murmur is common. (C, D) Severe aortic regurgitation: The length of the diastolic murmur is variable. With preserved left ventricular function (C), the murmur usually is pandiastolic and medium frequency (high velocity, large volume reflux). The systolic murmur may be very prominent and long in duration, even in the absence of aortic stenosis. If there is left ventricular failure or the late end-diastolic pressure is markedly elevated, resulting in a narrow gradient between the aorta and left ventricle during the last third of diastole, the diastolic murmur may be short and unimpressive (D). The systolic murmur also may be unremarkable in this setting; this combination can result in a serious underestimation of the severity of aortic regurgitation.

trivial or very mild AR may be so short as to be little more than a blurring sound off A_2. Such murmurs typically are of low amplitude and high frequency and hard to hear without selective focus on early diastole. With increasing degrees of aortic reflux, the murmur may become truly holodiastolic but remains decrescendo in quality

(Figures 12-5B and 12-5C). Therefore, in a patient with a diastolic blood pressure of 60 mmHg or less, a pandiastolic murmur would be anticipated. Some patients with *severe* aortic regurgitation actually may have a *shorter* decrescendo diastolic murmur than those with milder disease (Figure 12-5D). "Free" aortic regurgitation commonly is associated with a very high, late left diastolic ventricular filling pressure and a low aortic diastolic pressure. This results in a small aortic-left ventricular gradient in late diastole so that the amount of reflux may be small or nil at end diastole (see Figure 12-5D).

Intensity

The aortic regurgitation murmur ranges in loudness from very faint to quite prominent but rarely is of grade 4–5/6 intensity and only occasionally has an associated thrill. Trivial degrees of aortic regurgitation produce murmurs that typically are soft. It is important not to miss such a faint murmur, as the presence of audible AR supports the diagnosis of organic heart disease. Echocardiography confirms that trivial to mild AR commonly is inaudible.

Although the amplitude of the diastolic murmur roughly correlates with severity, some persons with a small degree of aortic leak have a loud murmur. Patients in heart failure resulting from severe aortic regurgitation occasionally have no more than a faint, short murmur. Severe AR actually can be silent.

Optimal Sites for Auscultation

The murmur of aortic regurgitation usually is heard best adjacent to the sternum between the second and fourth left interspace. In mild or trivial AR, the murmur may be localized only to the second left interspace at the left sternal edge. With increasing severity, the maximal intensity of the murmur may be as low as the fourth or fifth interspace. The murmur often is audible at the apex when its intensity is grade 2–3/6 or more, and in some subjects it actually may be heard best at the apex. This finding is more likely to occur in elderly patients.

Aortic Regurgitation Heard to the Right of the Sternum

The typical aortic regurgitation murmur may be heard easily at the second to third right interspace where it can be quite prominent. However, the murmur is usually not detectable lower down the right side of the sternum. Many years ago, Levine and Harvey observed that, on occasion, an aortic regurgitation murmur is very well heard at the *lower right sternal border* (3rd to 5th right interspace). They noted that this phenomenon occurred commonly in patients who had *disease of the aortic root* rather than at the valve level.

Conditions that result in an aortic regurgitation murmur heard best on the right side of the sternum include:

- Aortic aneurysm (idiopathic or due to cystic medial necrosis or syphilis)
- Sinus of Valsalva aneurysm
- Aortic dissection (acute or chronic)
- Selective perforation or eversion of the right coronary cusp

Aids to Auscultation

Special techniques are not necessary to increase audibility of a loud regurgitant murmur. However, the elusive, faint, high-pitched blowing murmur of AR can be made more audible by certain maneuvers. In some cases, these maneuvers may be necessary to hear the murmur. The optimal method of auscultation is as follows. The examination should take place in a quiet room with the patient sitting, standing, or leaning forward with the breath held in mid- or full expiration. Use firm pressure with the diaphragm of the stethoscope (enough to leave an imprint on the skin). Background noise, such as that from air conditioning or the patient's own breath sounds, can readily mask detection of a high-pitched, grade 1–2/6 aortic murmur. When there is a question or no murmur is heard but there is reason to believe that aortic regurgitation is present, the use of sustained handgrip or squatting may "bring out" a faint murmur. Both maneuvers increase systemic resistance and central aortic pressure and can augment the degree of aortic reflux.

In some patients, particularly younger persons, the AR murmur may be heard more easily in the supine position. Remember that in older adults, especially those with chronic lung disease or congestive heart failure, the AR murmur may be maximal or heard only at the LV apex, which can be misleading.

Systolic Murmur

A systolic ejection murmur is common in moderate to severe aortic regurgitation. It results from an abnormally large stroke volume ejected with rapid force often across an anatomically deformed aortic valve into an enlarged proximal aorta. *Practical Point: A loud systolic murmur in a patient with severe aortic regurgitation does not necessarily imply coexisting aortic stenosis.* Typically, this systolic murmur is short and peaks before the second half of systole if there is no aortic valve obstruction (see Figures 12-5B and 12-5C). However, with a large ejected stroke volume, the systolic murmur lengthens in proportion to the increase in left ventricular ejection time. Thickened aortic valve leaflets may accentuate the intensity and duration of the systolic murmur. Severe aortic regurgitation without stenosis rarely may be associated with a grade 4/6 systolic murmur and an accompanying thrill.

Associated Valve Lesions

Patients can have both aortic stenosis and regurgitation, particularly with rheumatic disease. In these instances, the systolic murmur also reflects the aortic valve obstruction. Typically, this results in a prominent systolic *and* diastolic murmur, the so-called bellows murmur. When both the systolic and diastolic murmurs are long, this combination may mimic a continuous murmur along the left sternal border.

When mitral stenosis coexists with AR, the obstruction to inflow to left ventricular filling may attenuate the full expression of the aortic regurgitation on clinical examination. The diastolic murmur of AR may be less prominent and evidence for LV dilatation less impressive than that usually produced by a comparable degree of aortic regurgitation.

Austin Flint Murmur

The Austin Flint murmur (AFM), a well-known auscultatory phenomenon, is a low-pitched, rumbling apical diastolic murmur that sounds exactly like the murmur of mitral stenosis (see Figures 12-4 and 12-6). Its presence generally indicates a large diastolic leak with a regurgitant fraction of over 50%. The AFM usually is found in association with the peripheral signs of severe AR (see Table 12-1). It is important to correctly identify the AFM for the following reasons: (1) its presence indicates that the aortic reflux is severe and (2) accurate identification of the AFM on physical examination usually means that associated mitral stenosis is not present.

Pathogenesis

Many theories have been advanced to explain the Austin Flint murmur. The mechanism appears to be related to an incomplete opening of the anterior leaflet of the mitral valve during diastole as a result of the impact of the regurgitant stream of blood into the left ventricular cavity. The mitral valve closing motion in middiastole is more rapid than usual in patients with an AFM. The first vibrations of the Austin Flint murmur occur while the mitral valve leaflets are rapidly moving toward the left atrium as antegrade blood from the atrium transverses the narrowing but still open mitral valve orifice. The resultant low-

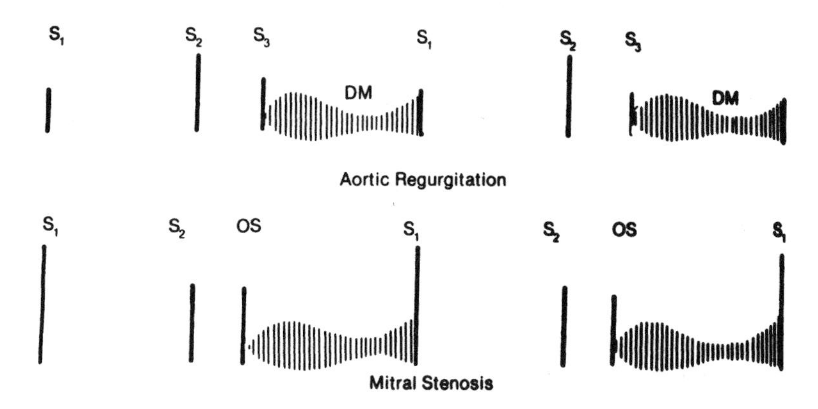

Figure 12-6. Similarity between the Austin Flint murmur of aortic regurgitation and the diastolic rumble of mitral stenosis. Both diastolic murmurs (DM) are low frequency and sound similar to each other. They are best heard using the bell of the stethoscope with light pressure at the left ventricular apex with the patient in left lateral position (see Figure 6-3). The Austin Flint murmur usually is accompanied by a soft S_1 and prominent S_3. The latter may be palpable, as may presystolic distention of the ventricle (S_4). The rumbling murmur of mitral stenosis classically is associated with an accentuated S_1 and a high-frequency opening snap (OS), which occurs closer to S_2 than does the S_3. In spite of these associated points, it may be exceedingly difficult to differentiate one murmur from the other.

pitched murmur may persist into late diastole as a result of turbulence within the left ventricular cavity. A late, presystolic murmur occasionally is part of the Austin Flint complex and actually may be the dominant diastolic component (see Figure 12-4). Typically, the AFM is found in patients with a greatly increased LV end-diastolic volume and a very large aortic regurgitant fraction.

Auscultatory Features

The Austin-Flint bruit is a rumbling diastolic murmur that usually begins in early to middiastole (see Figures 12-4 and 12-6). If a presystolic component is present, one will hear a crescendo, low-frequency murmur in late diastole that extends to the S_1. The pitch of the AFM is identical to the rumble of mitral stenosis. Typically, the murmur begins with a prominent S_3, and in many instances, the S_3 and the AFM fuse to produce an explosive initiation of a middiastolic rumble (see Figure 12-4).

Austin Flint or the Diastolic Murmur of Mitral Stenosis?
Patients with rheumatic heart disease frequently have combined aortic regurgitation and mitral stenosis. Therefore, it is important to accurately identify the etiology of a low-frequency, apical diastolic murmur in any patient with evidence of moderate to severe aortic regurgitation (see Figure 12-6). Evidence of associated mitral valve disease implies that the rumble is due to organic mitral stenosis and not secondary to severe aortic incompetence. Table 12-2 lists a number of differentiating features.

Differential Diagnosis

Pulmonary Regurgitation

In severe pulmonary hypertension, a high-pitched, blowing murmur is common (Graham Steell's murmur). Its acoustic characteristics are identical to those of mild aortic regurgitation. Graham Steell's murmur invariably is associated with other signs of pulmonary hypertension, such as a right ventricular lift and increased P_2.

Mitral Stenosis

Occasionally, the diastolic murmur of mitral stenosis is of medium to high frequency and may simulate aortic regurgitation if it radiates well to the lower left sternal border. Careful auscultation should identify a clear-cut interval between A_2 and the onset of the mitral stenosis murmur; an opening snap and an increased S_1 typically are present. If the opening snap is close to A_2 and the mitral stenosis murmur long

Table 12-2. Helpful Differentiating Features of an Apical Diastolic Murmur in Aortic Regurgitation: Austin Flint Murmur versus Mitral Stenosis

	Austin Flint	Mitral Stenosis
Rhythm	Normal sinus	Atrial fibrillation
Left ventricular heave	Common	Absent
Right ventricular lift	Absent	Present
S_1	Normal to decreased	Loud
Opening snap	Absent	Present
S_3	Present	Absent

and loud, one can be readily misled as to the murmur origin. Tachycardia accentuates this confusion.

Acute Aortic Regurgitation

In recent years, the unusual syndrome of acute massive aortic regurgitation increasingly has become recognized. Often this is a dramatic, life-threatening condition resulting from the sudden influx of an excessive amount of blood into a left ventricle unable to accommodate the large regurgitant volume. In such cases, the aortic valve usually is normal or only mildly abnormal prior to the onset of the sudden regurgitation. Acute or subacute bacterial endocarditis, aortic dissection, aortic valve perforation or rupture secondary to trauma, or myxomatous degeneration are the most common causes of this syndrome.

A prompt and accurate diagnosis of acute AR is of great importance as urgent surgical intervention usually is mandatory. However, the typical physical signs of severe chronic aortic regurgitation often are absent in such patients, and the aortic regurgitation murmur itself may be unimpressive in these severely ill patients (Table 12-3). Why is this so?

1. The voluminous regurgitant volume often precipitates acute left ventricular failure, with secondary systemic vasoconstriction and tachycardia. The arterial tree "clamps down," preventing or attenuating the classic blood pressure alterations and peripheral signs of chronic severe aortic regurgitation.
2. Sinus tachycardia is common in acute AR. The increase in heart rate results in a relative shortening of diastole, which hampers accurate auscultation by making identification of systole and diastole difficult.
3. Because the left ventricle usually is of normal thickness and diameter prior to the onset of the acute AR, it is nondistensible and unable to dilate. Left ventricular filling pressure becomes markedly elevated, and early to mid-LV diastolic pressure rises excessively. This rise results in premature closure of the mitral valve. S_1 is soft and there is no S_4 or presystolic component to the Austin Flint murmur. In these patients, left ventricular function often is acutely depressed. The tremendously elevated left ventricular pressure in late diastole causes a shortening of the AR murmur, often surprisingly soft and short because of a low cardiac output and decreased late diastolic aortic-LV gradient.

Table 12-3. Features of Acute versus Chronic Severe Aortic Regurgitation

	Chronic	Acute
Resting heart rate	Normal	Sinus tachycardia common; easy to confuse systole for diastole
Blood pressure	Increased systolic BP (>140 mmHg) Decreased diastolic BP (<70 mmHg) Increased pulse pressure	Normal or slight reduction in systolic BP; diastolic BP may or may not be low Pulsus alternans
Peripheral pulses	Bisferiens contour Increased amplitude and volume Peripheral signs of severe AR	Can have unremarkable contour with little or no evidence for peripheral vasodilatation
Jugular venous pulse	Normal	Mean pressure may be elevated V wave if functional tricuspid regurgitation
Precordial motion	LV impulse at fifth/sixth ICS, left anterior axillary line-hyperdynamic or heaving Contour Palpable S_3 or S_4 common	Normal or slight LV enlargement Bifid diastolic impulse with palpable S_3, sustained late diastolic motion RV impulse if severe pulmonary hypertension
Heart sounds	S_1 normal or decreased S_2 often unremarkable; increased to decreased A_2 S_3 very common S_4 uncommon Ejection click possible	S_1 decreased or absent S_2 single, soft or absent A_2, increased P_2 S_3 "always" S_4 common Ejection sound common Middiastolic mitral valve closure sound

Aortic regurgitation murmur	Medium frequency Usually holodiastolic May be short, with rapid decrescendo Grade 3 unless CHF present	Medium frequency, often harsh Musical if ruptured cusp Usually not holodiastolic, may be very short, rapidly decrescendo Can be quite soft
Austin Flint murmur	Common middiastolic component, with or without presystolic murmur	"Always" middiastolic component, with or without presystolic murmur
Systolic murmur	Typically present Can simulate aortic stenosis or mitral regurgitation	Typically present Mitral regurgitation murmur common

Physical Findings

The physical examination in acute aortic regurgitation may be dramatically different from a patient with chronic aortic regurgitation (see Table 12-3).

General Appearance

Patients with acute aortic regurgitation frequently are seriously ill and may be in acute heart failure. Resting tachycardia and orthopnea are common. The skin may be pale, cool, and moist, reflecting intense sympathetic vasoconstriction.

Blood Pressure and Pulses

The low diastolic blood pressure common to severe, chronic aortic regurgitation may be absent. The small forward stroke volume and decreased rate of ejection in these patients prevents the expected increase in systolic blood pressure. Therefore, the pulse pressure may be normal, slightly increased, or wide. The nonauscultatory signs of severe AR in the peripheral circulation may be unimpressive or totally absent, in contradistinction to chronic AR of an equivalent degree. A bisferiens pulse usually is not present.

Jugular Venous Pulse

Right ventricular failure resulting from pulmonary hypertension is common in severe acute AR. The jugular venous mean pressure often is elevated and tricuspid regurgitation may be present, resulting in large V waves in the neck veins (see Chapter 16).

Precordial Motion

The left ventricular impulse may be unimpressive in recent-onset aortic incompetence or displaced laterally with a thrusting contour. The greatly enlarged left ventricular impulse typical of chronic aortic regurgitation is absent if there has been no prior cardiac involvement. A right ventricular or parasternal impulse may be present if pulmonary artery pressure is elevated because of acute left ventricular failure.

Heart Sounds

S_1 is soft or even absent due to the premature closure of the mitral valve (see Figure 12-4). S_2 may be normal or single. Either or both S_3 and S_4 commonly are noted.

Aortic Regurgitation Murmur

The murmur of acute AR may be unimpressive, thus clinically misleading. If congestive heart failure or severe depression of LV function is present, the diastolic AR murmur may be soft. Frequently, severe aortic regurgitation produces a murmur with medium- to low-frequency vibrations, and the length of the murmur may be surprisingly short. If the acute AR is related to preexisting aortic root disease or isolated rupture of the right coronary cusp, the diastolic murmur may radiate best down the right sternal edge (see pages 172–173).

Austin Flint Murmur

The AFM commonly is found in acute aortic regurgitation, where it is likely to be middiastolic with or without a presystolic component (see Figure 12-4).

Systolic Murmur

The systolic flow murmur commonly heard in severe chronic AR also may be present in acute AR. If left ventricular function is depressed, this murmur is likely to be soft and short. Frequently, a long systolic murmur suggestive of mitral regurgitation is heard at the apex.

13

Mitral Regurgitation

In its various forms, mitral regurgitation is the most diverse of all acquired valvular lesions. The functional anatomy of mitral valve closure is complex; abnormal valve function may result from disease or distortion of the mitral leaflets, the valvular suspensory or supporting "apparatus," or the left ventricle itself. In addition, a number of pathologic conditions can affect the mitral valve, making mitral regurgitation the most common valve lesion in adults. In contradistinction to the other major valve disorders, the presence of mitral regurgitation may be acute, transient, or chronic and the subsequent hemodynamic sequelae may wax and wane in severity.

Normal Anatomy and Function

The mitral valve has two major leaflets or cusps: a large anterior or aortic leaflet and a smaller posterior or mural leaflet (Figure 13-1). The anterior leaflet is much broader in depth than the posterior and very mobile. The triscalloped posterior cusp comprises two thirds of the circumference of the mitral valve annulus; it is relatively narrow and is more limited in motion than the anterior leaflet. The surface area of leaflet tissue is two to three times greater than the area of the functional mitral orifice, providing ample margin for systolic coaptation that prevents reflux of blood into the left atrium.

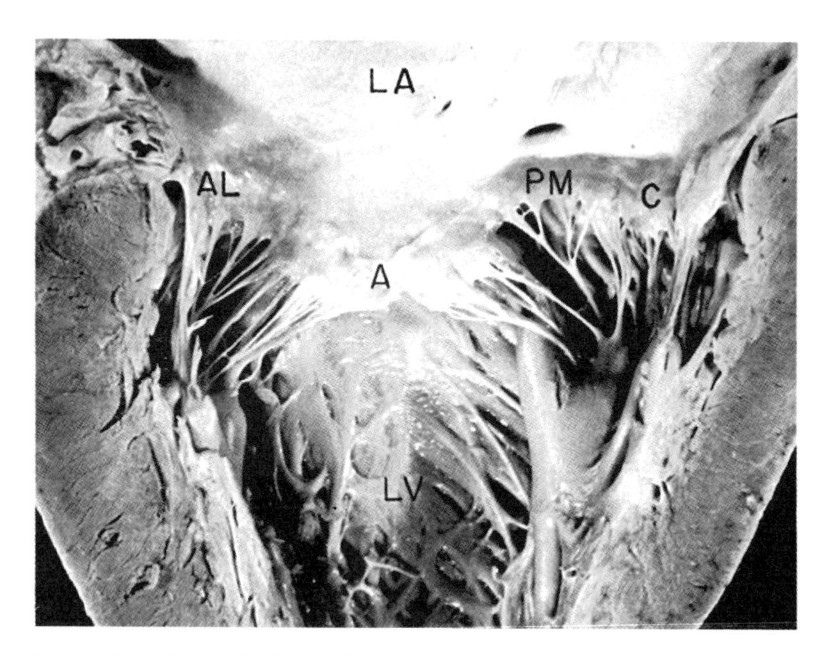

Figure 13-1. Normal mitral valve. This is an autopsy specimen of a patient with a normal heart. Note the complexity of the chordae tendineae and their fine structure. AL, PM, and C are the scallops of the posterior leaflet. AL = anterolateral, PM = posteromedial, C = central, A = anterior mitral leaflet, LA = left atrium, and LV = left ventricle. (Reprinted with permission from Lucas RV, Edwards JE. The floppy mitral valve. *Curr Probl Cardiol.* 1982;7:1.)

The two mitral cusps are anchored by a complex network of chordae tendinae, which insert at or near the free edges of the leaflets and also attach to the commissural aspects of the valve (see Figure 13-1). Most of the chordae arise from either of the two major papillary muscles in a cascading network of individual chords. The chordae are smooth, delicate strands of connective tissue and vulnerable to stretching, thickening, foreshortening, and rupture. The papillary muscles essentially are specialized extensions of the LV muscular trabeculae: There is an anterolateral and a posteromedial papillary muscle. *Practical Point: The posteromedial papillary muscle is more vulnerable to fibrosis, contraction, or rupture, probably because it has a less well-developed coronary blood supply than the anterolateral papillary muscle.* The two main papillary muscles have two to four separate heads, each giving rise to large first-order chordae tendinae. Each papillary muscle and its respective chordal attachments provide support to *both* the anterior and posterior valve leaflets.

During left ventricular isovolumic systole, the papillary muscles begin to develop tension as soon as intraventricular pressure rises and the mitral valve cusps move toward their final closing position. The apposing mitral leaflets bulge convexly toward the left atrium as the papillary muscles and chordae tauten during the remainder of systole. The leaflets themselves do not normally extend above the plane of the mitral valve annulus during ejection. Tension on the papillary muscles is greatest in mid- to late systole, when LV size has diminished substantially and the leaflets are prevented from excessive protrusion into the left atrium.

In early diastole, the mitral valve leaflets swing down into the LV during ventricular filling, quickly return to a closed position in mid-diastole after rapid filling, and are reopened by left atrial contraction. The mitral valve leaflets move rapidly to their final closed position following atrial contraction.

Functional and Anatomic Causes

Mitral regurgitation may have a variety of causes (Table 13-1), each relating to specific derangements of valvular or ventricular anatomy. The major etiologies of mitral regurgitation are discussed in greater detail later in this chapter.

Pathophysiology

The effects of an incompetent mitral valve on cardiac size and function are modulated by two factors: the *severity* of the mitral leak itself and the *duration* of the underlying hemodynamic disturbance. Mild mitral regurgitation produces relatively little derangement in left ventricular function. Moderately severe mitral regurgitation, when chronic, is surprisingly well tolerated for years. Major mitral regurgitation, particularly when acute or of recent onset, is poorly tolerated and frequently results in profound clinical deterioration. In general, the pathophysiology and compensatory changes are related more closely to the severity and duration of the valvular leak than to the underlying etiologic process.

Table 13-1. Major Causes of Mitral Regurgitation

Disorders of mitral valve leaflets
Rheumatic valvulitis, acute or chronic
Floppy valve syndrome
Mitral valve prolapse, some variants
Bacterial endocarditis
Disorders of papillary muscles
Ischemic heart disease, dysfunction rupture
Fibrosis
Cardiomyopathy
Aortic valve disease
Hypertensive heart disease
Lateral migration
Gross cardiac dilatation
Disorders of chordae tendineae
Floppy valve syndrome
Rupture
Idiopathic
Endocarditis
Disorders of mitral annulus
Calcification
Marked dilatation; for example, floppy valve syndrome

The Holosystolic Murmur

In patients with a classic holosystolic murmur of mitral regurgitation, reflux of left ventricular blood into the left atrium begins immediately with the rise in LV intracavitary pressure (Figure 13-2). Some studies have shown that up to 50% of the entire regurgitant volume may reflux into the left atrium *before* the aortic valve opens. *Therefore, the systolic murmur begins with the first heart sound.* The large left ventricular-left atrial pressure gradient during systole causes regurgitation to continue throughout ejection; the resultant murmur vibrations are heard up to and occasionally even beyond the aortic closure sound (A_2).

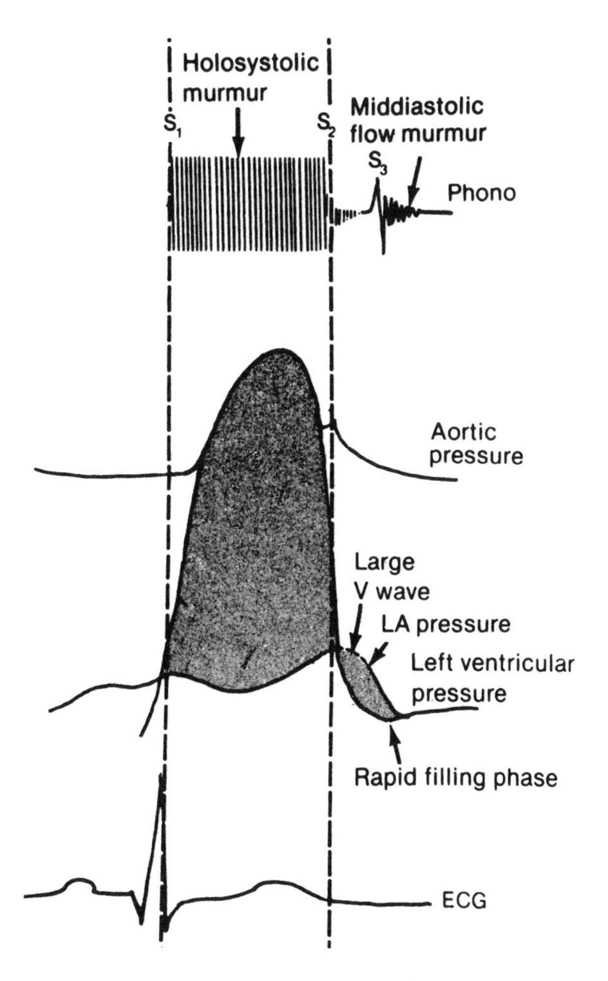

Figure 13-2. Pressure-sound correlations in mitral regurgitation. There is a large pressure gradient between the left ventricle and the left atrium that begins before the aortic valve opens and ends during isovolumic relaxation. This pressure difference results in a holosystolic murmur with sound vibrations beginning with S_1 and extending to S_2. The murmur classically is even or plateaulike in configuration, although many variants exist. An S_3 frequently is present when there is a significant degree of mitral regurgitation; the S_3 reflects the excessive blood volume traversing the mitral valve in early diastole. Such voluminous left ventricular filling may produce a short mid-diastolic flow murmur in patients with severe mitral regurgitation.

Left Ventricular Alterations

In severe mitral regurgitation, the regurgitant fraction (regurgitant volume divided by stroke volume) is over 50%; that is, more than half the LV stroke volume regurgitates back into the left atrium. The LV enlarges in response to the volume overload. During diastole the ventricle receives the blood refluxed into the left atrium *in addition to* the normal venous return from the right heart transmitted across the pulmonary circulation.

Most mitral regurgitant flow occurs before the middle of systole, as the LV "unloads" its large end-diastolic volume more rapidly than normal. Stroke volume usually is well preserved until late in the course of chronic, severe mitral regurgitation; LV ejection fraction is well maintained for a long period. In chronic mitral regurgitation, left ventricular and left atrial compliance increases, resulting in relatively low intracardiac filling pressures in spite of large intracardiac volumes. In long-standing rheumatic mitral regurgitation, severe elevation of left atrial pressure or significant pulmonary hypertension is unusual. Left atrial dilatation can be enormous and predisposes to atrial fibrillation.

LV function deteriorates relatively late in the course of severe mitral regurgitation. Once LV function becomes depressed, LV ejection fraction falls and end-diastolic and end-systolic volumes increase further; ventricular compliance decreases and LV filling pressure rises. Usually, the result is pulmonary congestion at rest or with relatively mild effort.

Acute Mitral Regurgitation

When acute mitral regurgitation results in abrupt or rapid-onset volume overload of the left heart, the preexisting size and compliance of the left atrium are paramount in determining the resultant signs and symptoms. A large volume of regurgitation into a normal, noncompliant atrium results in high left atrial pressures. The LV does not adequately tolerate an acute volume load when compensatory mechanisms of dilatation and hypertrophy lack time to develop; left ventricular diastolic and left atrial pressures increase markedly. The clinical course of such patients may decline rapidly. The physical examination often is considerably altered from those in chronic mitral regurgitation (see pages 217–220).

Physical Findings

Practical Point: Abnormalities of the carotid and jugular venous pulse, as well as precordial motion, are similar in all types of mitral regurgitation and related directly to the severity of the valvular leak. Therefore, the following discussion of these physical findings is pertinent to *all causes* of mitral regurgitation. However, characteristics of the systolic murmur and associated heart sounds vary considerably among the different types of mitral regurgitation.

Chronic rheumatic mitral valve disease is the prototype for all varieties of mitral regurgitation. In rheumatic mitral valvulitis, fibrosis and distortion of the valve tissue result in thickened, deformed cusps and chordae tendinae that may not function normally. Frequently, there is an element of commissural fusion, resulting in associated mitral valve stenosis. Dilatation of the cardiac chambers (both the left atrium and left ventricle) develops over a *prolonged* time.

Carotid Arterial Pulse

In mild mitral regurgitation of any etiology, the arterial pulse is normal. However, with moderate to severe regurgitation, the carotid pulse may be brisk or jerky, often with a decreased pulse volume. This results from a normal to decreased forward stroke volume that is ejected more rapidly than normal during early systole. The carotid pulse in severe regurgitation may be quick rising, poorly sustained, and low amplitude; it has been called a *small water-hammer pulse*, reminiscent of aortic regurgitation. *Practical Point: A small, quick arterial pulse in a patient with pure mitral regurgitation suggests that the valvular leak is hemodynamically important.*

Jugular Venous Pulse

There are no characteristic abnormalities of the venous pulse in mitral regurgitation unless right heart failure has occurred. Patients with severe mitral regurgitation and pulmonary hypertension often have functional (and occasionally organic) tricuspid regurgitation. In such instances, large jugular venous V waves that increase with inspiration will be seen.

Patients with chronic rheumatic mitral valve disease frequently are in atrial fibrillation; in this case, the venous A wave disappears and the V wave becomes more prominent, even in the absence of tricuspid regurgitation.

Precordial Motion

Left Ventricular Impulse

Mitral regurgitation typically produces a hyperdynamic apical impulse (see Chapter 4) with an increased amplitude and relatively brief and normal outward motion (Figure 13-3A). In chronic mitral regurgitation, the left ventricular apex beat is displaced laterally and downward as the LV enlarges. Pure mitral regurgitation rarely causes massive cardiac enlargement. With the development of abnormal LV function, the dilated LV takes on a more spherical or globular shape and the apical impulse may become sustained.

A systolic apical thrill will be felt when the systolic murmur is loud (grade 4/6 or greater). An early diastolic outward impulse commonly is detectable in severe mitral regurgitation; this can be subtle and may be appreciated best when the patient holds his or her breath in mid-expiration (see Figure 13-3A). The motion is the tactile component of the LV rapid filling wave; that is, a palpable S_3. A palpable A wave (S_4) never is found in chronic rheumatic mitral regurgitation.

Parasternal Impulse

There are several causes of a palpable lower sternal lift or impulse in patients with mitral regurgitation (Table 13-2). In severe mitral incompetence without significant pulmonary hypertension, the large regurgitant jet may reflux into the left atrium and produce a palpable outward recoil of the anterior cardiac structures (Figure 13-4). In such cases, careful palpation will reveal a brief, *late systolic impulse* beneath the lower sternum. This outward movement is *asynchronous* with the apical LV impulse occurring just *after* the apex beat is felt. The typical chest wall motion is a slow-rising, late-peaking systolic impulse that collapses in early diastole (Figure 13-3B).

More commonly, the parasternal impulse is related to pulmonary hypertension that results in *sustained* right ventricular lift (Figure 13-3C). High pulmonary artery pressures result in right ventricular hypertrophy and dilatation. In rheumatic heart disease, severe pulmonary hypertension is found most commonly in *combined* mitral

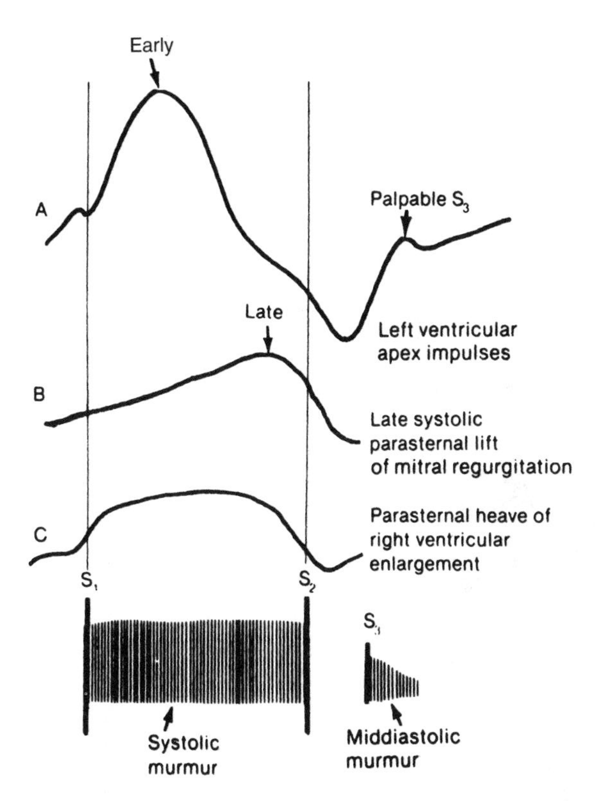

Figure 13-3. Precordial motion patterns in mitral regurgitation. (A) The left ventricular impulse is hyperdynamic with a normal contour and increased amplitude of the early systolic outward motion. A palpable third heart sound may be felt in the left decubitus position. In severe chronic mitral regurgitation, the left ventricular impulse may be sustained and heaving in quality (not diagrammed). B and C represent parasternal (right heart) activity. (B) A late systolic parasternal lift. This reflects an anterior thrusting motion of the heart that occurs in late systole. It is produced by regurgitation of a large volume of blood into an enlarged left atrium (see Figure 13-4). This late systolic lift is asynchronous with the left ventricular apical impulse, which is early systolic (see A). (C) Sustained parasternal lift. The most common finding in severe mitral regurgitation is a gentle holosystolic outward impulse palpable at the lower left sternal region. This usually is the result of pulmonary hypertension and right ventricular enlargement.

Table 13-2. Causes of Systolic Parasternal Lift in Mitral Regurgitation

	Cause
Late systolic	Large regurgitant jet into dilated left atrium
Holosystolic	Pulmonary hypertension with right ventricular hypertrophy
Holosystolic	Associated mitral stenosis

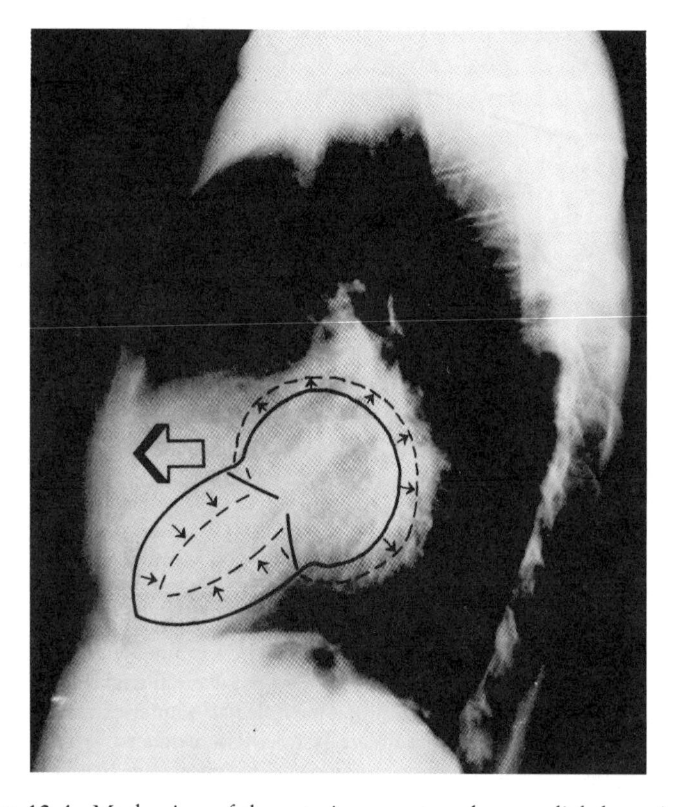

Figure 13-4. Mechanism of the anterior parasternal precordial thrust in severe mitral regurgitation. During systole a large regurgitant volume fills a dilated left atrium, thrusting the right ventricle forward. This results in palpable anterior displacement of the lower left sternal border, which is late systolic in timing and can be felt as a separate and delayed impulse when compared with simultaneous palpation of the left ventricular apex beat (see Figure 13-3). (Reprinted with permission from Abrams J. Precordial palpation. In: Horwitz LD, Groves BM, eds. *Signs and Symptoms of Cardiology*. Philadelphia: JB Lippincott Co.; 1985.)

regurgitation and stenosis and less frequently in pure mitral regurgitation. Other clues to pulmonary hypertension usually are present, including a palpable pulmonic ejection sound, loud P_2, and a right ventricular S_4. The murmur of tricuspid and pulmonary regurgitation also may be present, particularly the former.

Heart Sounds

First Heart Sound

Alterations in the intensity of S_1 are common in mitral regurgitation but of no diagnostic significance. The most frequent abnormality is a *decrease* in S_1 amplitude. A loud systolic murmur beginning with the rise of LV pressure may mask or blur identification of S_1. If there is associated mitral stenosis, S_1 may be normal or increased in intensity. A loud S_1 may be heard in holosystolic prolapse of the mitral valve (see Chapter 15).

Second Heart Sound

S_2 is unremarkable in mild to moderate mitral incompetence. In more severe cases, S_2 becomes audibly split in expiration and widely split during inspiration. *Practical Point: Prominent expiratory and inspiratory splitting of S_2 suggests hemodynamically significant mitral regurgitation and a large regurgitant fraction.*

P_2 is frequently accentuated in moderate to severe mitral regurgitation due to pulmonary hypertension.

Third Heart Sound

A third heart sound is common in mitral regurgitation of hemodynamic importance and implies a large regurgitant fraction (see Chapter 6). *Practical Point: An S_3 in severe mitral regurgitation often is related to the large volume of blood returning to the LV in early diastole and does not necessarily indicate left ventricular failure.* The S_3 occurs 0.12–0.20 sec after A_2 and may be quite loud. Its presence excludes mitral stenosis of more than an insignificant degree. Frequently, the S_3 can be felt in early diastole as a palpable, rapid-filling wave, particularly when the patient is turned to the left lateral recumbent position.

If congestive heart failure or LV dysfunction is present, the S_3 may reflect impaired cardiac function with LV dilatation. In this setting, the presence of an S_3 does not necessarily indicate a large regurgitant fraction. Therefore, detection of an S_3 in a subject with mitral regurgitation means one of two things: (1) a major mitral leak with a large regurgitant fraction and good ventricular function or (2) a diseased LV with a depressed ejection fraction.

Middiastolic Murmur

The S_3 in mitral regurgitation often is followed by a short middiastolic rumble or murmur (MDM) that represents reverberations from rapid and excessive filling of a distended left ventricle (see Figure 13-3C). *Practical Point: The presence of an S_3 and middiastolic murmur indicates severe mitral regurgitation in the absence of coexisting mitral stenosis.*

The MDM is a brief, low- to medium-pitched apical diastolic rumble best heard with the bell of the stethoscope when the patient is in the left decubitus position. It should be sought carefully in all patients with mitral regurgitation. It is critical to focus on the timing and the length of the MDM, as it is readily confused with the diastolic murmur of mitral stenosis. In pure mitral regurgitation, the MDM does not extend into late diastole. If related to mitral regurgitation, the S_3 will be a low-pitched thud and the MDM will end well before S_1. Carotid massage may be used to slow the heart rate to help make a more accurate auscultatory judgment.

Fourth Heart Sound

An S_4 of LV origin never is a feature of rheumatic mitral valve disease. The left atrium in chronic mitral regurgitation of any etiology usually is dilated, overly compliant, and unable to generate an atrial sound or S_4. This is in contradistinction to *acute* mitral regurgitation, where the normal-sized atrial chamber has very high pressure and increased volume; the left atrium contracts more forcefully than normal, typically producing an audible S_4. A right ventricular S_4 may be present in patients with severe pulmonary hypertension who are in sinus rhythm; inspiratory augmentation and maximal intensity at the lower sternal edge suggest an S_4 of right-sided origin.

Opening Snap

Contrary to popular belief, an opening snap occasionally may be present in patients with pure rheumatic mitral regurgitation (see page 227). This probably relates to thickened, stiff, and distorted mitral leaflets. The opening snap coincides with the opening motion of the anterior leaflet.

The presence of an audible opening snap raises the question of coexisting mitral stenosis. In such cases, the intensity of S_1 and the presence and length of the diastolic rumble require special attention.

Murmur of Rheumatic Mitral Regurgitation

The typical murmur of mitral regurgitation is a constant-amplitude systolic murmur beginning immediately with S_1 and extending to S_2. It usually is of medium-high frequency, heard best at the LV apex, and radiates clearly into the left axilla.

Length and Shape

In rheumatic mitral regurgitation, a central jet of blood usually refluxes into the left atrium, producing a sound vector that extends posteriorly and laterally. Regurgitation begins during isovolumic systole and extends into the isovolumic relaxation phase. Therefore, the murmur is typically holo- or pansystolic with an even intensity throughout systole (see Figures 13-2 and 13-5A).

In auscultation of systolic murmurs, concentration on the last third of systole is important (see Figure 8-4). Does the murmur extend to S_2? Is there a sound gap or murmur dropout before A_2? *Practical Point: In almost all cases of mitral regurgitation, sound vibrations in late systole continue until S_2, although the murmur may have a variable contour.* Occasionally, the murmur of mitral regurgitation appears to begin just *after* S_1. This may be due to masking of audible sound by S_1 or very low-amplitude murmur vibrations in early systole.

The murmur of rheumatic mitral regurgitation may taper or augment in late systole. The most common variant is mid- to late-systolic accentuation of the murmur. Sound vibrations may fan out during the last third of systole (Figure 13-5B). Such a murmur, similar to that of papillary muscle dysfunction or mitral valve prolapse, is typical of mild mitral reflux. In more severe mitral regurgitation, the murmur is more likely to have midsystolic accentuation, giving it a spindle-shaped or ejection quality (Figure 13-5C). In all these situations, careful auscultation usually will identify sound vibrations at the *beginning* and at the *end* of systole, which confirm that the murmur truly is regurgitant in quality as opposed to a more common systolic ejection murmur.

The least common variant of the mitral regurgitation murmur is one that tapers or decreases in intensity in late systole (Figure 13-5D and Table 13-3). This configuration also is more likely to be found in

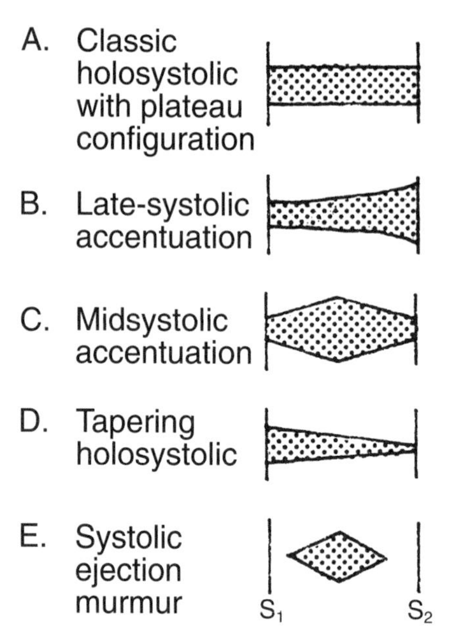

Figure 13-5. Variable contours of the murmur of mitral regurgitation. A through D represent holosystolic murmurs with differing configuration (see the text); note that sound vibrations extend to S_2 in each example. (E) A typical systolic ejection murmur is shown for comparison. Note the sound-free interval immediately following S_1 and, most important, at the end of the murmur.

Table 13-3. Causes of Late-Systolic Tapering of the Murmur of Mitral Regurgitation

Mild or trivial degree of mitral regurgitation
Recent or acute onset mitral regurgitation (giant V wave)
Severe mitral regurgitation with relatively small left atrium (giant V wave)
Improved mitral valve coaptation resulting from decreased LV cavity size in late systole

trivial degrees of mitral regurgitation; the murmur usually is very soft. In such cases, the major question for the observer is whether the murmur is truly holosystolic. This may be exceedingly difficult to resolve. In severe, recent-onset mitral regurgitation, the murmur often is decrescendo in late systole due to the enormous left atrial V wave and a decrease in late-systolic reflux into the atrium (Figure 13-6). The murmur may take on ejection characteristics (Figure 13-5E). Such attenuation in late systole does not occur in chronic rheumatic mitral regurgitation.

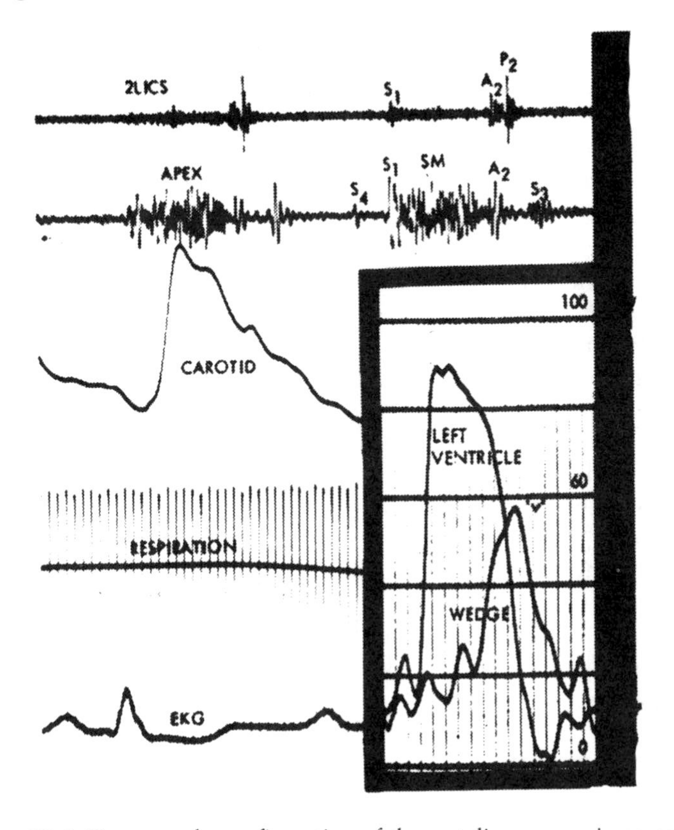

Figure 13-6. Decrescendo configuration of the systolic murmur in severe mitral regurgitation. This postinfarction patient has mitral regurgitation and congestive heart failure. Cardiac catheterization (lower right) reveals an enormous V wave in the pulmonary capillary wedge tracing, consistent with severe mitral regurgitation. Because of the rapidly diminishing pressure gradient between the left ventricle and the left atrium in late systole, the murmur decreases in intensity during the last part of systole. Therefore, the murmur of severe mitral regurgitation, particularly when of recent onset, may take on ejection characteristics. Note the presence of an S_3 and S_4, common in severe acute mitral regurgitation. (Reprinted with permission from Reddy PS, Shaver JA, Leonard JJ. Cardiac systolic murmurs: Pathophysiology and differential diagnosis. *Prog Cardiovas Dis.* 1971;14:1.)

Intensity

In general, the louder the murmur of rheumatic mitral regurgitation is, the greater the degree of reflux. Patients with a moderate to severe mitral leak and a large regurgitant fraction usually have grade 3–4/6 systolic murmurs. Therefore, a systolic apical thrill is common in severe mitral regurgitation. However, there are important exceptions to this rule: Certain conditions predispose to a murmur of decreased amplitude even when the regurgitation is major. On occasion, the murmur may be barely audible in the setting of severe regurgitation. *Practical Point: The most important factor affecting murmur intensity is the state of left ventricular function. With preserved LV contractility and vigorous systolic function, the velocity and volume of blood flow is high and the murmur is loud. If LV dysfunction occurs and the LV ejection fraction falls, the murmur will become softer, even though the degree of mitral incompetence remains unchanged.* Many patients with severe mitral regurgitation and a soft murmur are in overt congestive heart failure. With appropriate medical therapy, LV function may improve: End-diastolic volume decreases, ejection fraction increases, and the murmur becomes louder. In profound pump failure and end-stage mitral regurgitation, the systolic murmur may be virtually inaudible. This situation is more likely to occur in acute (nonrheumatic) mitral regurgitation, such as severe papillary muscle dysfunction or rupture in acute myocardial infarction in association with marked depression of myocardial performance.

Under the following conditions, the intensity or loudness of the mitral regurgitation murmur will be decreased out of proportion to the degree of reflux:

- Congestive heart failure or left ventricular dysfunction
- Low cardiac output states
- Associated mitral stenosis
- Hugh left atrium
- Large right ventricle
- Obesity
- Chronic obstructive lung disease
- Thick muscular chest

In the last three conditions, all intracardiac sound tends to be diminished.

The most common cause of a soft murmur is a trivial degree of mitral regurgitation. The intensity of the murmur of mitral incompetence does not vary with changes in cycle length (e.g., in atrial fibrillation, post-PVC beats). Typically, the murmur retains its baseline loudness, irrespective of cycle length. This is in contradistinction to ejection or flow murmurs, which augment in intensity following a long diastolic filling period.

Experience with Doppler echo indicates that *acoustically silent* mitral regurgitation, especially mild to moderate, commonly is download in many patients.

Frequency or Pitch

In mild degrees of mitral reflux, the LV-LA gradient is high, the amount of regurgitant blood is relatively small, and the flow velocity is high; the resultant murmur is high pitched. Firm pressure with the diaphragm of the stethoscope routinely should be used in auscultation for mitral regurgitation. An apical, high-pitched holosystolic murmur is a common finding in a young person with mild mitral regurgitation with a prior history of acute rheumatic fever. Typically, on physical examination, no other abnormalities will be present.

With increasing degrees of reflux, the left atrial "V wave" increases in size as the gradient between the left ventricle and the left atrium decreases. This change produces a murmur with lower-frequency vibrations. In many patients with a substantial degree of mitral regurgitation, the murmur has mixed frequencies, reflecting both a large gradient and high flow. The typical mitral regurgitation murmur has a whirring, somewhat musical pitch. In severe mitral regurgitation, the murmur may be harsh in quality.

Location and Radiation

Mitral regurgitation of any etiology is appreciated best at the left ventricular apex, although on unusual occasions the murmur will be heard better elsewhere over the chest. In some individuals, the murmur may be louder just inside the apex impulse; in tall, thin subjects with small hearts, the murmur and apical impulse can be medial, near or adjacent to the left sternal edge. The murmur of chronic, rheumatic mitral regurgitation rarely is heard best away from the PMI. However, in some cases of isolated rupture of chordae tendinae with selective or dominant incompetence of the posterior leaflet, the murmur actually may be maximal at the first or second left interspace (see pages 215–216). The classic rheumatic murmur radiates leftward into the axilla and often is heard well at or beneath the left scapula in the posterior chest. When the left atrium is large, the murmur may be audible over the thoracic vertebral column.

Left Decubitus Position

Practical Point: Auscultation in the left recumbent position (see Figure 14-3) *usually will augment the murmur of mitral regurgitation and often increase its intensity by one to two grades. In addition, this maneuver occasionally accentuates the holosystolic nature of a late, tapering murmur. Use this position routinely when an apical systolic murmur is of low amplitude and long duration.*

Occasionally, loud mitral regurgitant murmurs radiate rightward and are heard readily at the lower sternal border. These murmurs may occur in patients with large left ventricles; in such cases, one must be sure there is no coexisting tricuspid regurgitation. In patients with small hearts, the murmur of mitral regurgitation may be medial, with poor radiation into the axilla due to interpositioning of the lungs. With marked enlargement of the right ventricle, the palpable apex beat may not be formed by the LV and the mitral regurgitation murmur may be heard best in the left axilla *lateral* to the apparent apical impulse. With a markedly dilated LV, the murmur may be louder in the axilla than at the apex. Unless posterior leaflet incompetence is prominent, the murmur of mitral regurgitation does not radiate well to the base of the heart.

The murmur of mild mitral regurgitation is not only soft but often well localized to a small area of the precordium at or near the apex. Selective listening or tuning in for this faint, high-pitched murmur is important. Auscultation while the patient's breath is held in mid- or end expiration is helpful in identifying these soft murmurs.

Middiastolic Rumble

A brief diastolic, low-frequency rumble at the apex, following a loud S_3, is common in severe mitral regurgitation (see Figures 13-2 and 13-3) and has been discussed already (see page 194). It is important to remember that such a murmur does not necessarily indicate associated mitral stenosis. This murmur is heard best using light pressure with the bell of the stethoscope precisely positioned on the apex beat. The left recumbent position is essential, as often the middiastolic murmur cannot be detected at any other site or position.

Assessment of Severity

Table 13-4 lists various findings on physical examination that suggest hemodynamically significant chronic mitral regurgitation.

Differential Diagnosis of the Systolic Murmur of Mitral Regurgitation

The murmur of mild mitral regurgitation readily can be mistaken for an *ejection murmur* with apical radiation, particularly if the mitral murmur is decrescendo in quality. The critical question relates to the *length* of the murmur in late systole. An apical murmur that is crescendo or fans out to S_2 invariably is some form of mitral regurgitation. Attention to post-PVC beats may be of aid in this differential diagnosis; ejection murmurs augment in intensity, whereas the loudness of the mitral regurgitation murmur remains unchanged.

Tricuspid regurgitation may be a difficult problem to separate from mitral regurgitation when there is significant right ventricular enlargement. In this setting, the apical murmur actually may arise from the right heart and reflect tricuspid regurgitation. Careful attention to

Table 13-4. Bedside Clues to Hemodynamically Severe Chronic Mitral Regurgitation

Rhythm: Many patients are in atrial fibrillation
Carotid pulse: Small volume, quick rising
Left ventricular impulse: Hyperdynamic, forceful, often displaced to left; may be sustained; systolic apical thrill common
Parasternal impulse: Early or late systolic (in absence of mitral stenosis)
S_2: Widely split; increase P_2
S_3: Present, may be palpable; middiastolic "flow" rumble often audible
Murmur: Usually very loud; if CHF present, murmur often becomes louder after successful therapy

respiratory variation is essential. The tricuspid murmur usually, but not always, increases during inspiration, but the murmur of mitral regurgitation typically softens with inspiration. Unfortunately, some tricuspid regurgitation murmurs do not vary with respiration. If there is associated atrial fibrillation, respiratory changes in murmur intensity may be virtually undetectable.

A *ventricular septal defect* murmur can simulate mitral regurgitation, although its maximal location at the lower sternal border should readily differentiate the two. However, in patients with small hearts or long chests, the mitral regurgitation murmur can be medial. In all three causes of a holosystolic murmur (mitral regurgitation, tricuspid regurgitation, and ventricular septal defect), the murmur may be decrescendo in late systole and can simulate a systolic ejection murmur. Mitral regurgitation, as opposed to the other lesions, typically is heard *best* at the apex and usually will have some radiation to the axilla.

In *hypertrophic cardiomyopathy*, mitral regurgitation commonly is present. A long systolic ejection murmur is typical in these patients, and it often is difficult to be sure that there is a *separate* murmur of mitral regurgitation. The typical radiation pattern of the regurgitant murmur often is absent in hypertrophic cardiomyopathy. Careful assessment of the response of the systolic murmur to positional changes, maneuvers, and pharmacologic agents may be helpful (see Table 11-1).

Papillary Muscle Dysfunction

A variety of conditions leading to fibrosis, ischemia, or contractile dysfunction of the papillary muscles and the surrounding left ventricular muscle can result in mitral regurgitation. Papillary muscle dysfunction commonly is responsible for mitral regurgitation associated with coronary artery disease.

Pathophysiology

Normal function of the papillary muscles helps prevent the mitral valve leaflets from protruding into the left atrium during systole. As the size of the left ventricular cavity decreases during ejection, the mitral valve cusps and chordae are held firmly in place by the two contracting papillary muscles (Figure 13-7A). Tension generated by

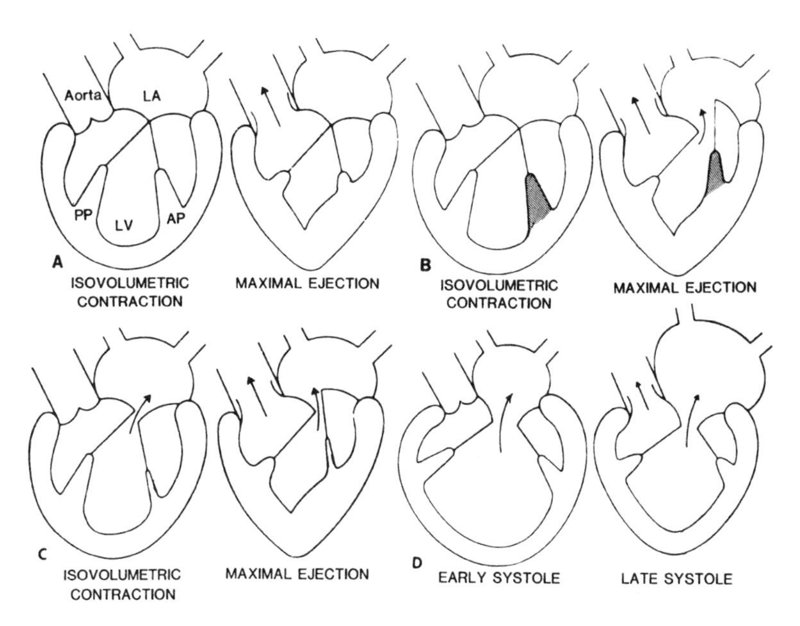

Figure 13-7. Mechanisms of mitral regurgitation caused by papillary muscle dysfunction. (A) In a normal heart, the papillary muscles contract during systole as left ventricular cavity size diminishes. An intact mitral apparatus prevents reflux of blood from the ventricle into the left atrium. (B) In the papillary muscle dysfunction shown here, the posterolateral papillary muscle is functionally abnormal (ischemia or infarction) and unable to maintain valvular apposition during peak systole when the left ventricular cavity size is at its nadir. The mitral leaflet(s) protrudes into left atrium and mid- to late-mitral regurgitation occurs. The mitral valve typically remains competent in early systole; therefore, there is no murmur during the first third of systole. (C) In this example of papillary muscle scarring, the papillary muscle is so fibrotic or atrophic that even during isovolumic systole it is unable to prevent reflux of blood into the left atrium because of an inadequate tethering effect on the chordae tendineae. The mitral regurgitation may worsen during ejection. (D) In this example of a markedly dilated left ventricle, the papillary muscles are displaced laterally and lose their normal alignment within the left ventricular cavity. This may result in inability of the mitral valve to adequately coapt because of abnormal tension on and displacement of the mitral valve apparatus. The resultant murmur of mitral regurgitation is believed to be related to distortion of papillary muscle-ventricular anatomy rather than true dysfunction. (Reprinted with permission from Burch GE, DePasquale MP, Phillips JH. The syndrome of papillary muscle dysfunction. *Am Heart J*. 1968;75:399.)

the papillary muscles is maximal in *late systole*, when LV dimensions are smallest. When abnormal structure or function alters papillary muscle contraction, the mitral leaflets may prolapse, resulting in reflux of blood into the left atrium typically during the last half of systole (Figures 13-7B and 13-7C). Therefore, the classic murmur of papillary muscle dysfunction is a *late-systolic crescendo murmur* extending up to S_2 (Figure 13-8A). When there is severe contractile dysfunction or marked fibrosis and shortening of the papillary muscles, the resultant mitral regurgitation may be *holosystolic*; however, in such situations the murmur often retains late-systolic accentuation (Figure 13-8B). Papillary muscle murmurs often have midsystolic accentuation and take on ejection characteristics (Figure 13-8C).

Myocardial ischemia is the most common cause of papillary muscle dysfunction. The posteromedial papillary muscle is especially vulnerable because its blood supply usually is scant and its collateralization is poorer than that of the anterolateral papillary muscle. In humans, the papillary muscles *and* adjacent left ventricle often are found to be scarred or necrotic at autopsy. The murmur of papillary muscle dysfunction commonly may be heard during acute myocardial infarction and rarely may be observed during attacks of angina pectoris.

Patients with considerable fibrosis in the left ventricle from any cause frequently have a mitral regurgitation murmur that may result from abnormal papillary muscle function. Severe LV wall motion abnormalities or an overt ventricular aneurysm is likely to involve one of the papillary muscles (the posteromedial most commonly), resulting in mitral regurgitation.

Many different disease processes can cause scarring or damage to the papillary muscles (Table 13-5). Myocardial fibrosis can result from severe left ventricular hypertrophy of any cause. Moderately severe left ventricular dilatation also may result in mitral regurgitation related to the papillary muscles. In such patients, the papillary muscles are pulled laterally away from their normal alignment in the left ventricular cavity and lose the optimal angle for generation of wall tension, producing prolapse of the mitral valve leaflets (Figure 13-7D). This proposed mechanism has been disputed by some experts.

Papillary Muscle Rupture

When acute transmural myocardial infarction causes complete rupture of the body or tip of a papillary muscle, it typically involves the

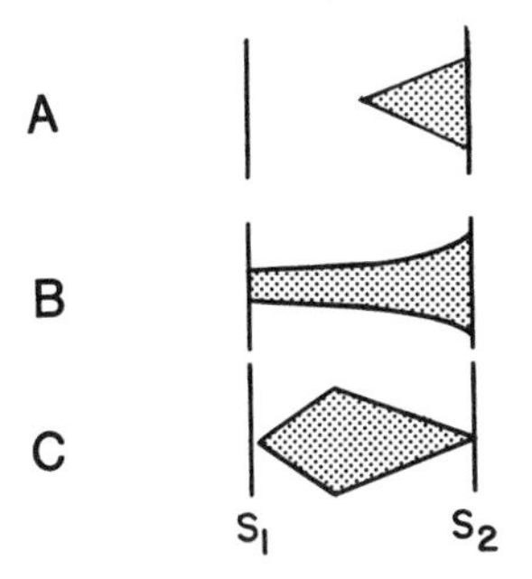

Figure 13-8. Configuration of papillary muscle murmurs. (A) In the classic late systolic contour, the mitral valve leaflets remain competent in early systole. (B) In a holosystolic murmur with late systolic peaking or accentuation, the papillary muscle is unable to sustain valve competency throughout systole; when the ventricle reaches its minimal size, mitral reflex increases and the murmur becomes louder. (C) An ejection-shaped murmur may occur due to a very large left atrial V wave resulting in a late systolic decrease in mitral regurgitation (see Figure 13-6). Another proposed mechanism for the decrescendo murmur of papillary muscle dysfunction is improvement in late systolic leaflet coaptation due to the decrease in late systolic left ventricular cavity size.

posteromedial muscle. In this situation, the degree of mitral regurgitation is massive and usually fatal. A flail mitral leaflet results from profound disruption of the mitral supporting apparatus. The resultant syndrome of acute mitral regurgitation (see pages 217–220) is a true emergency and these patients can be saved only by surgical treatment.

Physical Examination in Papillary Muscle Dysfunction

Carotid Pulse

There are no specific abnormalities of the carotid pulse. With severely depressed LV function and a low cardiac output, the amplitude of the pulse wave will be small and mechanical alternans may be detectable (see Chapter 2). If the mitral regurgitation is severe, the carotid pulse may be quick rising and of low amplitude, producing a soft tapping impulse under the palpating finger.

Table 13-5. Etiologies of Papillary Muscle Dysfunction

Dysfunction	Etiology
Ischemic heart disease	Miscellaneous
Acute myocardial infarction	Carcinoid heart disease
Angina pectoris (transient)	Vasculitis
Healed myocardial infarction	Myocarditis
Left ventricular aneurysm	Endocardial fibroelastosis
Left ventricular fibrosis	Abscess
Left ventricular dilatation	Trauma
Congestive cardiomyopathy	Amyloid
Hypertrophic cardiomyopathy	Endocarditis

Jugular Venous Pulse

No abnormalities of the venous pulse are present in papillary muscle dysfunction unless there is biventricular congestive failure, in which case the mean venous pressure will be elevated.

Precordial Motion

Because the majority of patients with a papillary muscle dysfunction murmur have left ventricular dysfunction or dilatation due to underlying coronary artery disease, the apex impulse often is abnormal (Table 13-6). An ectopic precordial impulse may be present, suggesting left ventricular aneurysm or a severe localized abnormality of wall motion. More commonly, a palpable S_4 (presystolic distention of the left ventricle) will be noted (see Figure 6-2). If the mitral leak is large and left ventricular diastolic volume excessive, a palpable rapid filling wave (S_3) may be detected. A bifid apical thrust or a sustained or late systolic lift consistent with deranged LV function may be present.

When there is severe mitral regurgitation, a late systolic parasternal impulse reflecting left atrial expansion in systole occasionally can be felt (see Figures 13-3B and 13-4).

Heart Sounds

First Heart Sound

The first heart sound is soft, normal, or increased in papillary muscle dysfunction and therefore of little diagnostic help. Frequently, an S_1 of increased intensity is found in such patients.

Table 13-6. Precordial Motion Abnormalities Commonly Associated with Papillary Muscle Dysfunction

LV heave (sustained)
Bifid or double LV apical impulse
LV impulse displaced laterally
Ectopic LV impulse
Palpable S_4
Palpable S_3
Late parasternal lift

Second Heart Sound

S_2 is unremarkable in the majority of cases of papillary muscle dysfunction. S_2 may show abnormally wide splitting if there is severe mitral regurgitation (see Chapter 5). Ischemic dysfunction of the left ventricle or left bundle branch block may produce reversed splitting of S_2 in the setting of a papillary muscle dysfunction murmur. If there is pulmonary hypertension, P_2 will be increased in intensity.

Third Heart Sound

An audible and even palpable S_3 is a common accompaniment of papillary muscle dysfunction. This sound may result from a large volume of blood crossing the mitral valve in diastole if the mitral regurgitant fraction is large. The S_3 also may be related to left ventricular dysfunction and increased left ventricular diastolic pressure and volume; other evidence of heart failure is common in this situation.

Fourth Heart Sound

A prominent S_4 or atrial gallop typically is found in association with papillary muscle dysfunction. Underlying left ventricular dysfunction is associated with a high left ventricular end-diastolic pressure and increased myocardial stiffness. The S_4 may be extremely loud and often is palpable in the left decubitus position. *Practical Point: The absence of an S_4 in the setting of a late-systolic murmur suggests the murmur is not due to papillary muscle dysfunction.*

Systolic Murmur

The hallmark of papillary muscle dysfunction is an apical, medium-high frequency systolic murmur that begins well after S_1, usually in midsystole, and fans outward to S_2 (see Figures 13-8A and 13-9). The murmur typically is soft, usually of grade 2/6 intensity, and may wax and wane with serial observation.

Shape and Duration

Papillary muscle murmurs have many configurations, which include early decrescendo, midsystolic, pansystolic, and late systolic (see Figure 13-9). *Practical Point: The classic murmur configuration of papillary dysfunction has its onset in early to midsystole, with sound vibrations extending up to S_2.* The murmur may or may not appear to begin with S_1. If LV contractility is preserved, the murmur can be decrescendo in late systole, as LV cavity size decreases and the degree of late systolic mitral reflux diminishes. Frequently, the configuration of the murmur varies, being ejection quality one day and holosystolic the next. Major mitral regurgitation due to papillary muscle dysfunction produces a pansystolic murmur that often has late systolic accentuation (see Figure 13-8B) but may be diamond shaped (see Figures 13-5C and 13-8C).

Intensity and Frequency

The murmur of papillary muscle dysfunction usually is not prominent, although with severe mitral regurgitation (as with papillary muscle rupture), the murmur can be loud. Considering the actual degree of the valvular leak, the murmur commonly is soft, particularly in acute myocardial infarction, where the pump function of the ven-

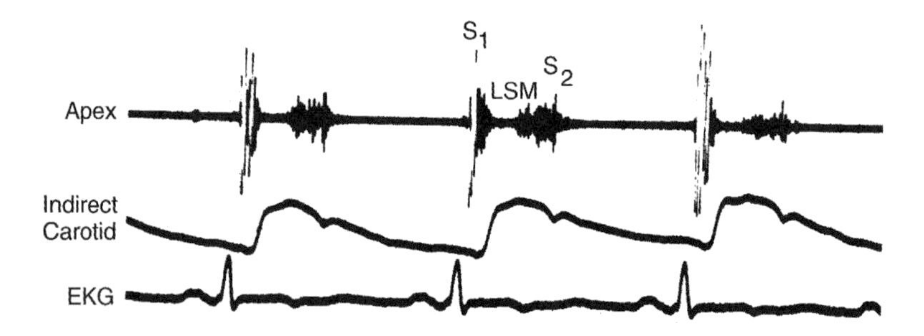

Figure 13-9. The classic late-systolic murmur in a patient with coronary artery disease. This subject had mild mitral regurgitation at angiography. (Reprinted with permission from Reddy PS, Shaver JA, Leonard JJ. Cardiac systolic murmurs: Pathophysiology and differential diagnosis. *Prog Cardiovasc Dis.* 1971;14:1.)

tricle may be profoundly depressed. In papillary muscle dysfunction, the relationship between murmur intensity and the severity of mitral regurgitation typically is poor, due to the coexistence of serious abnormalities of left ventricular contraction. Cases of truly silent, severe papillary muscle dysfunction or rupture with major mitral regurgitation have been documented. *Practical Point: Be careful not to underestimate the potential hemodynamic significance of a soft papillary muscle dysfunction murmur in acute myocardial infarction. On occasion, profound mitral regurgitation can exist with a very faint (grade 1–2/6) systolic murmur.*

As left ventricular function improves, the murmur of papillary muscle dysfunction may either disappear or get louder as contractile force and ejection fraction increase. *Practical Point: Variability in the amplitude of the murmur is a common feature of papillary muscle dysfunction.*

The murmur of papillary muscle dysfunction usually is medium pitched, pure frequency in tone, and often has high-frequency components. Because these murmurs typically are soft, firm pressure with the diaphragm of the stethoscope is essential for optimal auscultation.

Location and Radiation

Usually, the murmur of papillary muscle dysfunction or rupture is maximal at the apex. Radiation patterns of the low intensity papillary muscle murmurs usually are unremarkable.

Papillary Muscle Dysfunction in Acute Myocardial Infarction

Careful, repetitive auscultation of patients with acute, transmural myocardial infarction will reveal an apical systolic murmur in 30–50% of patients. Both the intensity and shape are likely to change during the course of hospitalization. While often this murmur is ejection in nature at first, repeated listening may reveal holosystolic or late systolic vibrations. As a result of the decreased stroke volume and depressed ejection velocity that occurs in most patients with acute myocardial necrosis, typically a low-frequency, low-amplitude murmur is heard. *It is important to listen for this murmur in a very quiet setting, as it easily is missed.* In the case of a patient with an acute infarction, development of a new systolic murmur is common and likely to be heard within the first few days after admission. Infrequently, the murmur will retain its ejection quality, or it may have a purely late systolic accentuation that implies mild mitral regurgitation.

Papillary Muscle Rupture
This devastating but rare complication of acute myocardial infarction produces acute, severe mitral regurgitation. The murmur may be silent or very soft or loud and harsh. An S_4 and S_3 are common, and the patient is likely to be in acute pulmonary edema, with or without hypotension. Late systolic tapering of the murmur may be present as a result of a decreasing left ventricular-left atrial pressure gradient in end systole, produced by a huge left atrial V wave (see Figures 13-5D and 13-6).

Mitral Regurgitation Secondary to Left Ventricular Dilatation
Patients with cardiac decompensation or massive cardiomegaly often have a murmur of mitral regurgitation in the absence of intrinsic disease of the mitral valve. Frequently, the holosystolic murmur disappears or softens after treatment of congestive heart failure and clinical improvement. This murmur has been described as *functional* mitral regurgitation. It has been believed that the incompetent mitral valve results from dilatation of the mitral annulus. However, the mitral annulus does not always enlarge its circumference even in severe left ventricular enlargement. In the floppy mitral valve syndrome, the mitral ring or annular size consistently is found to be dilated.

The precise mechanisms for mitral regurgitation in dilated hearts remain controversial. Burch suggested that mitral regurgitation may result from malalignment and lateral migration of the papillary muscles in large ventricles, with the inadequate ability to tether the chordae at the appropriate tangent to the mitral valve orifice (see Figure 13-7D). In many patients with significant LV enlargement, the ventricular cavity becomes more spherical; the circumference of the dilated LV at midventricular level usually is larger than the annulus. The subsequent loss of normal papillary muscle geometry with respect to the long axis of the left ventricle could result in failure of the mitral valve apparatus to produce complete valve closure.

In these patients, the physical examination is similar to that of classic papillary muscle dysfunction; in addition to the holosystolic murmur, abnormalities of left ventricular precordial motion are likely to be found. Although this murmur may have late systolic accentuation, it typically fills systole.

Abnormalities of the Chordae Tendineae

The multiple thin chordae tendineae supporting the mitral valve become abnormally stretched and attenuated in various conditions;

rarely, a chord actually may rupture. The resultant mitral regurgitation ranges from mild to severe, depending on the number and location of the affected chordae, the preexisting status of the mitral valve, and the size and function of the left ventricle. The chordae to one or both leaflets may be involved. Often the supporting struts to one or two scallops of the posterior leaflet will rupture. If the ruptured chord is distal to the main truncal chordae and attached directly to the valve, the resultant valve deformity will be minimal. However, rupture of a proximal first or second order chord will cause major instability of the mitral cusp and significant mitral regurgitation.

Table 13-7 lists conditions associated with ruptured chordae tendineae. In patients with floppy mitral valve syndrome, mitral regurgitation may result from severe prolapse of the mitral leaflets caused by elongated but intact chordae or rupture of the abnormally thin chordae, producing sudden mitral incompetence. In the majority of cases, the posterior leaflet is involved. In such patients, the mitral valve annulus often is extremely dilated and the mitral leaflets are composed of excessive and redundant tissue. Recent surgical experience indicates that chordal rupture in subjects with myxomatous degeneration of the mitral valve is a common cause of severe mitral regurgitation.

Patients with rheumatic mitral disease usually do not undergo chordal rupture, perhaps because of the thickened, foreshortened subvalvular structures. Endocarditis can disrupt chordal function either in the setting of acute valve infection or months to years after bacterial eradication.

Table 13-7. Causes of Ruptured or Severely Stretched Chordae Tendineae

Idiopathic (spontaneous)
Infective endocarditis, acute and healed
Blunt chest or cardiac trauma
Myxomatous degeneration of the mitral valve ("floppy valve syndrome")
Marfan's syndrome
Previous myocardial infarction
Acute myocardial infarction with rupture of tip of the papillary muscle and chordae tendineae (rare)
Rheumatic mitral valvulitis
Vigorous physical effort (?)

The most severe sequelae of ruptured chordae tendinae are experienced in patients with a previously normal heart, in whom a major proximal chord ruptures suddenly, with resultant severe acute mitral regurgitation (flail mitral leaflet). The normal left ventricle and left atrium suddenly are presented with an acute, massive volume overload, resulting in excessively high intracardiac pressures. The left atrium and ventricle respond with vigorous and hyperactive contraction (Starling effect), often detectable on physical examination. Huge, left atrial V waves and increased left atrial pressure can result in severe pulmonary hypertension. Initially well tolerated, the mitral regurgitation typically results in dilatation and hypertrophy of the left atrium and ventricle over time; eventually, the mitral regurgitation converts to a more chronic hemodynamic state.

If the chordae to only one valve cusp are disrupted, only one of the mitral leaflets or scallops may protrude into the left atrium. The posterior leaflet is affected far more often than the anterior; an individual posterior scallop may prolapse by itself. On occasion, the portion of the valve that prolapses into the atrium produces a hoodlike deformity, which directs the regurgitant stream opposite to the site of valve prolapse (Figure 13-10). This "ectopic" jet of blood may produce unusual patterns of murmur radiation. Myxomatous alteration of the leaflet tissue and mitral valve prolapse usually underlie these cases of floppy valve syndrome.

Physical Findings in Ruptured Chordae Tendineae

In patients with ruptured chordae, the physical examination is influenced strongly by the presence or absence of preexisting structural heart disease. A heart that had been normal will present a picture of *acute mitral regurgitation* with no evidence of significant enlargement of the cardiac chamber. On the other hand, a patient with evidence of LV dilatation or atrial fibrillation is likely to have had *prior* mitral regurgitation. In this case, the diagnosis of a ruptured chordae tendineae may be based on the abrupt deterioration of the clinical picture or a change in the intensity of the preexisting murmur. Patients with ruptured chordae tendineae and a flail mitral leaflet have severely deranged hemodynamics and often are in overt congestive heart failure.

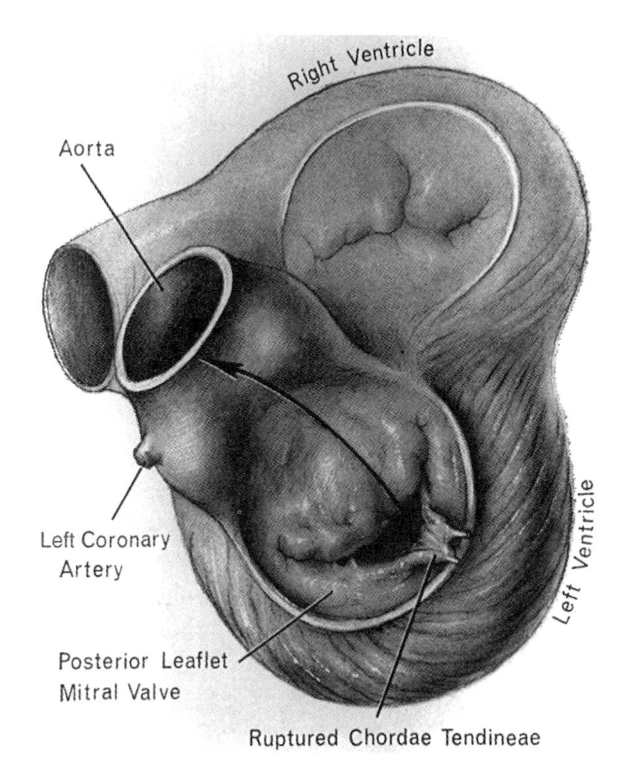

Figure 13-10. Ruptured chordae tendineae to the posterior mitral leaflet with subsequent selective posterior cusp insufficiency. The mitral regurgitation jet impinges on the medial aspect of the left ventricular outflow tract. This can produce a systolic murmur that radiates to the cardiac base. Posterior leaflet insufficiency is more common in an isolated rupture of the chordae tendineae, probably because the chordae to the posterior leaflet are thinner and less sturdy than those supplying the anterior leaflet. (Reprinted with permission from Selzer A et al. The syndrome of mitral insufficiency due to isolated rupture of the chordae tendineae. *Am J Med.* 1967;43:822.)

Carotid Pulse

If the degree of mitral regurgitation is large, the arterial pulses are likely to be quick rising with a rapid falloff. The pulse volume is normal to decreased. The rhythm almost always is regular (sinus) in patients with ruptured chordae unless there has been long-standing, mitral regurgitation and chronic atrial fibrillation.

Venous Pulse

There are no abnormalities of the jugular venous pulse unless pulmonary hypertension and right ventricular failure occur as a result of the acute massive volume overload. In such instances, the mean venous pressure will be elevated and large V waves of tricuspid regurgitation may be noted.

Precordial Motion

In a patient with no prior cardiovascular disease, the apex impulse will not be displaced laterally but will be exaggerated in amplitude (hyperkinetic) as a result of the acute volume overload. A palpable S_4 in the left recumbent position is common and its presence should be sought. *Practical Point: Detection of a palpable or audible* S_4 (see Figure 13-6) *confirms the presence of acute or recent-onset mitral regurgitation and virtually excludes a chronic rheumatic etiology.* With massive mitral reflux, a sustained right ventricular lift may be present at the lower left sternal border as a result of pulmonary artery hypertension. The recoil from the large regurgitant jet (huge left atrial V wave) may produce an anterior parasternal impulse confined solely to late systole (see Figures 13-3 and 13-4).

In patients with preexisting cardiac disease, LV enlargement is likely to have been present prior to the onset of chordal rupture. A sustained and displaced apex beat indicates previous cardiac enlargement or depression of LV function.

A visible and palpable S_3 often is present. Because the typical murmur of mitral regurgitation from ruptured chordae is loud, an apical systolic thrill may be present. If an eccentric regurgitant jet occurs as a result of posterior leaflet hooding, the transmitted thrill may be at the base or the second and third left interspace (see Figure 13-10). This would be an unusual site for the typical mitral regurgitation murmur.

Heart Sounds

First Heart Sound

There are no specific alterations in the first heart sound in ruptured chordae tendineae. S_1 may be soft if the P-R interval is long or loud if the anterior mitral leaflet is excessively mobile.

Second Heart Sound

Changes in S_2 in patients with ruptured chordae are similar to those in severe mitral regurgitation of any etiology. These include wide splitting of S_2 in expiration (shortened left ventricular systole) and an increased P_2 if pulmonary hypertension is present. A_2 may be lost in the loud holosystolic murmur, giving the appearance of a single second sound.

Third Heart Sound

Frequently, an S_3 is found in patients with ruptured chordae tendineae. The S_3 may be palpable and is coincident with the rapid filling wave that may usher in a short, middiastolic rumble.

Fourth Heart Sound

An atrial sound (S_4) coincident with a loud mitral regurgitation murmur is of great diagnostic importance, as it suggests the left atrium is contracting forcefully (see Figure 13-6). Often, the low-frequency S_4 is better felt than heard; careful palpation and auscultation while the patient is in the left recumbent position is mandatory. In such cases, the presence of an S_4 correlates with an elevated left ventricular end-diastolic pressure.

Mitral Regurgitation Murmur

Configuration and Duration

Since the mitral reflux caused by ruptured chordae tendineae usually occurs in the setting of a normal, noncompliant left atrium, a moderate to severe degree of regurgitation commonly will result in giant left atrial V waves and substantial elevation of atrial pressure. The LV-LA pressure gradient in late systole often is decreased because the actual amount of reflux into the left atrium decreases considerably in the latter third of systole (see Figure 13-6). This results in a tapering of sound vibrations and a decrescendo configuration to the murmur. Often, peak murmur intensity occurring in midsystole produces a crescendo-decrescendo systolic murmur. *Practical Point: Although the murmur of ruptured chordae tendineae commonly simulates a systolic ejection murmur, careful auscultation invariably will detect sound vibrations extending to* S_2. In fact, such a murmur often obliterates A_2.

Frequency and Intensity

Most patients with ruptured chordae initially have normal left ventricular function unless severe, preexisting heart disease is present. As the amount of the regurgitant volume is likely to be large, the murmur typically is loud (grade 3–4/6 intensity), often with an accompanying thrill. The murmur may be somewhat harsh compared to the more musical, whirring murmur of rheumatic mitral regurgitation.

Location and Radiation

Often chordal rupture causes eccentric localization and radiation of the murmur as the protrusion or hooding of one of the leaflets or scallops directs the regurgitant jet in a well-localized stream. Selective incompetence of the posterior leaflet or scallop resulting from chordal stretching or rupture tends to deflect the refluxing torrent of blood toward the medial left atrial wall and left ventricular outflow tract (see Figure 13-10). The sound vibrations radiate toward the proximal aorta, and the murmur may have its maximal intensity at the second left or right interspace. A preponderant deformity of the anterior leaflet directs the blood posterolaterally to produce a murmur that is loudest at the apex and left posterior thorax. The posterior leaflet is more likely to be involved in chordal rupture because its supporting chordae normally are thinner than those to the anterior cusp; in addition, the overall cuspal length is far greater than the anterior.

Mitral Regurgitation Masquerading as Aortic Stenosis

Posterior chordal rupture repeatedly has been documented to result in a loud murmur at the cardiac base (second or third interspace), simulating an aortic ejection murmur. This murmur may be maximal either at the aortic area or apex, but even in the latter case, it may be prominent at the base. Often the murmur appears to have a shorter duration at the aortic area. *Practical Point: When the murmur of a posterior ruptured chordae tendineae has a crescendo-decrescendo shape, it easily is mistaken for aortic stenosis. To avoid the error of confusing mitral regurgitation with aortic stenosis, pay attention to the length of the* systolic *murmur at both the aortic area and apex as well as to the quality of the carotid upstroke.*

Several large series of patients with ruptured chordae tendineae have demonstrated that there is no predictable or consistent relationship between the site of maximal murmur intensity and the specific leaflet involved. Clinicians should be aware of the vagaries of the clinical presentation of chordal rupture, particularly with respect to the false diagnosis of aortic stenosis.

Middiastolic Murmur

The large volume leak found in many of these patients will result in a middiastolic flow rumble (see Figures 13-2 and 13-3), usually initiated by an S_3. Its presence indicates involvement of a major degree of mitral regurgitation.

Acute Mitral Regurgitation

Acute mitral regurgitation is potentially a life-threatening condition. It therefore is important to understand the unique hemodynamics that produce a clinical picture different from that of chronic mitral regurgitation. Physicians should be alert to the important differences between the presentation of acute and chronic mitral insufficiency (Table 13-8).

Etiology

Severe *papillary muscle dysfunction* or *rupture* and *ruptured chordae tendineae* typically produce mitral regurgitation of acute or recent onset. *Endocarditis* is another cause of sudden mitral regurgitation; in this condition, the mitral valve leaflets can erode or perforate, or

Table 13-8. Differentiating Features of Severe Acute and Chronic Mitral Regurgitation

	Chronic	Acute
Rhythm	Often atrial fibrillation	Sinus rhythm or sinus tachycardia
Precordial examination	Hyperkinetic LV with lateral downward displacement	Hyperkinetic LV without lateral downward displacement
	LV heave possible; palpable S_3 often; apical thrill; can have parasternal or LA lift	Palpable S_3; palpable S_4; apical thrill frequently common; parasternal LA lift
Heart sounds	S_3 common, no S_4; OS occasionally noted; increased P_2 if pulmonary hypertension	S_3 and S_4 common; occasional OS (if posterior leaflet, especially with RCT); increased P_2
Systolic murmur	Typically holosystolic, even, whirring; may have mid- or late-systolic accentuation, maximum at apex	Typically loud, harsh murmur with late-systolic decrescendo; may appear to be ejection in quality; may be very prominent at aortic area or 2 LICS

infection can involve the supporting apparatus and result in rupture of a chord. Blunt or perforating *trauma* can result in acute mitral regurgitation if the mitral leaflets or supporting apparatus are damaged or disrupted.

Pathophysiology

In all cases of acute mitral regurgitation, the sine qua non is the sudden onset of severe reflux into a normal-sized left atrium. The full force of left ventricular systolic pressure is transmitted directly into a nonexpansile atrium, producing huge V waves. Left ventricular end-diastolic pressure increases and left atrial contractile force is enhanced. The left ventricular ejection rate and the LV ejection fraction actually may be higher than normal. Pulmonary capillary wedge and pulmonary arterial pressures increase, often dramatically. Severe pulmonary hypertension may ensue, and signs of right ventricular failure may appear.

As long as left ventricular systolic function is preserved, the increase in LV diastolic volume is vigorously ejected into both the aorta and left atrium; forward cardiac output typically is maintained despite a large regurgitant fraction. With time, LV mass and size increase, and this acute hemodynamic state may convert to the pathophysiology of chronic mitral regurgitation.

In some patients with severe acute mitral regurgitation, the clinical picture may be dramatic. The clinical course is far shorter, and early surgical intervention may be mandatory if LV function becomes deranged or pulmonary congestion severe. With the onset of overt congestive heart failure, the elevated systemic vascular resistance produced from reflex arterial vasoconstriction may worsen the hemodynamic situation by increasing the afterload of the left ventricle, thus increasing the degree of mitral regurgitation.

Physical Findings

At the time of examination, many patients are in mild to severe congestive heart failure and therefore may manifest orthopnea, tachypnea, and audible pulmonary crepitations (see Table 13-8). The heart rate usually is increased. The arterial pulse rises and collapses quickly as a consequence of severe mitral regurgitation, although the presence of congestive heart failure may sufficiently attenuate the pulse volume to preclude a meaningful assessment. The mean jugular venous pressure often is elevated; large A and V waves may be present. The latter will be dominant if there is associated tricuspid regurgitation caused by a high pulmonary artery pressure.

Precordial examination usually reveals a hyperdynamic left ventricular impulse, often with a palpable S_3. Unless there is preexisting cardiomegaly, the apex impulse will not be displaced laterally. Patients with papillary muscle dysfunction may demonstrate an ectopic left ventricular impulse or a sustained or bifid apical thrust. One hallmark of acute mitral regurgitation is the increased force of left atrial contraction producing an audible and often palpable S_4 (see Figures 6-2 and 13-6). Palpation in the left recumbent position is mandatory and may be more sensitive than auscultation in detecting the low-frequency S_4. An S_3 commonly is heard in severe acute mitral regurgitation (see Figure 13-6). Most subjects with acute or recent-onset mitral regurgitation have a large volume leak; the resultant vigorous left atrial expansion may produce an anterior thrust of the entire heart. This produces a late systolic parasternal lift (see page 190 and Figures 13-3 and 13-4).

As previously indicated, the murmur of acute mitral regurgitation may taper markedly in late systole and have a crescendo-decrescendo contour (see Figure 13-5), because the huge left atrial V wave causes near equilibration of the left ventricular-left atrial pressure in mid- to late systole (see Figure 13-6). If left ventricular function remains well preserved, the murmur will be loud, typically accompanied by a thrill.

Eccentric radiation patterns, especially with posterior leaflet incompetence, may produce a systolic murmur that is loudest at the second left interspace or aortic area and readily mimics aortic stenosis. The majority of murmurs of acute mitral regurgitation are loudest or equally loud at the apex; careful auscultation will demonstrate that the murmur is truly holosystolic. Some murmurs may end before S_2, which is consistent with an enormous left atrial V wave (see Figure 13-6). Typically, the murmur of a flail anterior mitral leaflet is loudest in the left posterior chest and may be heard along the vertebral column as well as at the top of the skull. In fact, many murmurs of acute mitral regurgitation can be heard over the entire thoracic vertebral column.

A short, middiastolic murmur that immediately follows S_3 is common in patients with severe mitral regurgitation of acute or chronic etiology. Its presence indicates a large regurgitant fraction. A separate holosystolic murmur along the lower sternal border, which increases with inspiration, indicates associated tricuspid regurgitation that may occur as a result of marked elevation of pulmonary artery pressure. Table 13-8 compares and contrasts some of the important diagnostic features of acute and chronic mitral regurgitation.

14

Mitral Stenosis

Mitral stenosis is a common sequela of acute rheumatic fever, found in as many as 40% of individuals with chronic rheumatic heart disease. Only half these patients can recall a prior history of an illness compatible with acute rheumatic fever.

Functional Anatomy and Pathophysiology

Chronic rheumatic valvulitis culminating in mitral stenosis is a result of thickening and distortion of the valve leaflets and chordae tendineae along with fusion and dense adherence of the mitral valve structures (Figure 14-1). Commonly, the process begins at the mitral valve commissures and may be limited to commissural fusion, resulting in a pliable valve that swings freely open, although the central orifice is narrowed. Typically, the leaflets are thickened and have blunted and rolled edges (Figures 14-1A, C). The chordae are foreshortened and often matted together. The entire valve apparatus becomes altered into a funnel-like sleeve; when severe, the mitral valve takes on a "fish mouth" appearance and loses the ability to open during diastole (Figures 14-1B, E). Dense calcification is a frequent late accompaniment.

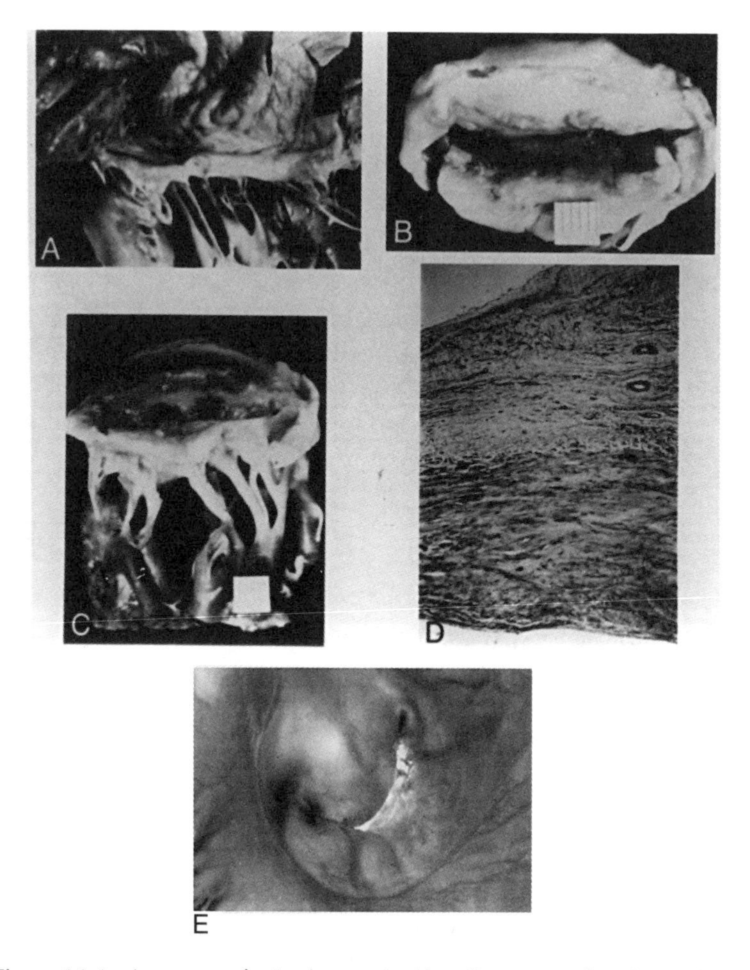

Figure 14-1. Anatomy of mitral stenosis. (A) Effacement of scallops of the posterior leaflet due to fusion of leaflet clefts. (B, C) Two views of a stenosed mitral valve removed at surgery. Note the commissural and cleft fusion in leaflets (B) and chordal changes (C). (D) Photomicrograph of mitral leaflet demonstrating sclerosis, vascularization, and nonspecific chronic inflammation. (E) Atrial view of a crescent-shaped stenotic orifice. Note the loss of individual scallop identity of the posterior leaflet. The anterior leaflet usually retains its shape and mobility until late in the disease process. This valve is transilluminated from the ventricular side; note the relative transparency of the anterior leaflet. (A–D: Reprinted with permission from Silver MD. *Cardiovascular Pathology*. New York: Churchill Livingstone; 1983:Vol. 1. E: Reprinted with permission from Beck AE, Anderson RW. *Cardiac Pathology*. New York: Raven Press; 1983.)

Relationship of Physical Findings to Pathologic Anatomy

The thickened and stiff mitral apparatus produces prominent sound transients as the mitral leaflets hinge open, then close during the cardiac cycle (Figure 14-2). The mitral closure sound (S_1) is accentuated, and the mitral valve opening motion, which is normally silent, results in a loud sound (opening snap) occurring as the fused valve cusps open abruptly into the LV cavity.

The dominant murmur of mitral stenosis consists of an early- to middiastolic murmur. In addition, a late-diastolic or presystolic murmur may occur, following left atrial contraction.

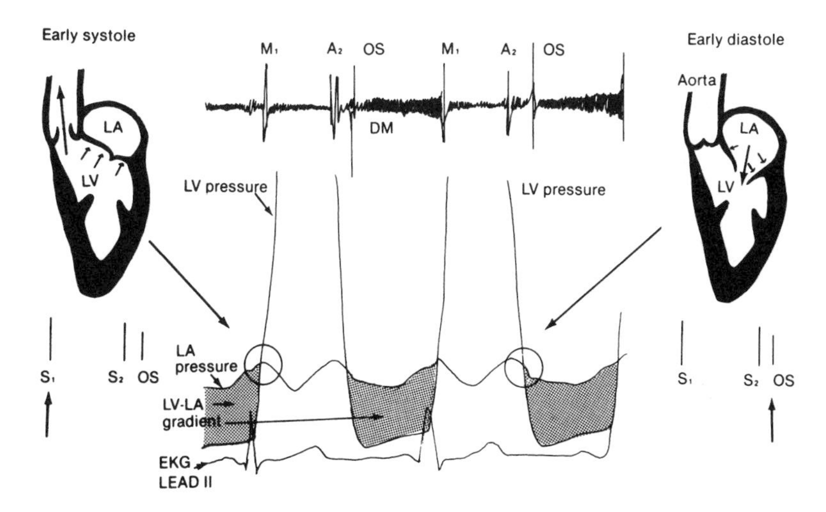

Figure 14-2. Intracardiac pressure and sound relationships in mitral stenosis. Pressure crossover between the left atrium (LA) and the left ventricle (LV) always precedes the cardiac sounds generated by mitral valve closure (M_1) and opening (opening snap). The persistence of a late diastolic gradient between the left atrium and left ventricle in combination with the thickened mitral valve apparatus results in an accentuated S_1. Similarly, the maximal opening excursion of the rigid and fibrotic valve generates an opening snap (OS), which immediately precedes early diastolic filling of the left ventricle and the resultant diastolic murmur (DM).

Clinical Spectrum

The normal mitral valve area is approximately 5 cm^2 (range 4–6 cm^2). Although physical signs (opening snap, short diastolic mumble) may be detectable in very mild mitral stenosis, symptoms usually do not appear until the mitral valve area has been reduced to at least 50% of normal (e.g., to 2–2.5 cm^2). When the mitral valve area is reduced to 1.5–2.0 cm^2, the mitral stenosis is mild to moderate and symptoms of fatigue and dyspnea are common.

Major hemodynamic sequelae occur when the valve area is reduced to 1.5 cm^2 or less, resting cardiac output may be depressed and LA pressure elevated. Often, relatively little effort may cause severe symptomatic limitation. When the mitral valve area is reduced to 1.0 cm^2 or less, severe or "tight" mitral stenosis is present. To maintain adequate flow at rest, the LA pressure often is elevated to 20–25 mmHg or greater.

Physical Examination

General Appearance

Most patients present no distinguishing features. Subjects with advanced mitral valve disease and right ventricular failure typically are thin and often have acrocyanosis and peripheral edema.

Jugular Venous Pulse

The venous pulse is normal in mitral stenosis unless there is associated atrial fibrillation, pulmonary hypertension, or right ventricular failure. Patients in sinus rhythm with elevated pulmonary artery pressure may show a prominent A wave in the venous pulse. Once RV decompensation ensues, mean venous pressure elevates. Tricuspid regurgitation, a common complication, results in a large systolic CV wave (see Chapter 16).

Carotid Arterial Pulse

The arterial pulse in mitral stenosis has a normal or decreased pulse volume and a normal contour. If the cardiac stroke volume is decreased, the carotid impulse will be diminutive; the finding of a small arterial pulse is common in patients with hemodynamically significant mitral stenosis.

Precordial Examination

Considerable clinical information can be derived from precordial examination in mitral stenosis. Typically, an increased S_1 amplitude is felt at or inside the site of the LV apex beat. An increased P_2 and, less commonly, a pulmonary artery lift may be felt at the second to third left interspace. The opening snap often is palpable in the region between the lower left sternal border and the cardiac apex. Careful timing of these palpable shocks is essential. The carotid and apical impulses are essential to aid in the identification of systole and diastole. A diastolic thrill at the apex, produced by a very loud mitral rumble, occasionally may be detected in the left decubitus position.

Left Ventricular Impulse

The left ventricle in pure mitral stenosis typically is underfilled and, therefore, does not produce a forceful apical impulse. It is essential to locate the LV apex beat to assist in optimal auscultation of the mitral diastolic rumble. This is done best in the left recumbent position (Figures 14-3A and 4-4). The PMI is normal or of decreased amplitude, nonsustained.

Right Ventricular Impulse

It is common to detect parasternal activity in pure mitral stenosis. Often this is manifest as a gentle, low-amplitude RV lift detectable at the third to fifth left interspace adjacent to the sternum. *Practical Point: To detect parasternal motion, it is desirable to use firm pressure with the heel of the hand during held expiration* (Figures 14-3B and 4-5). A right ventricular impulse often will be detected in mitral stenosis, even when resting pulmonary pressure is high normal or only moderately elevated. In individuals with more severe pulmonary hypertension, the RV impulse can be very prominent. The parasternal heave or major RV enlargement often extends leftward; in severe degrees of RV enlargement, the apex may be formed by the RV. The typical rumble of mitral stenosis may not be heard unless auscultation occurs when one listens precisely over the LV impulse, which may be displaced laterally in the anterior or midaxillary line by a huge RV.

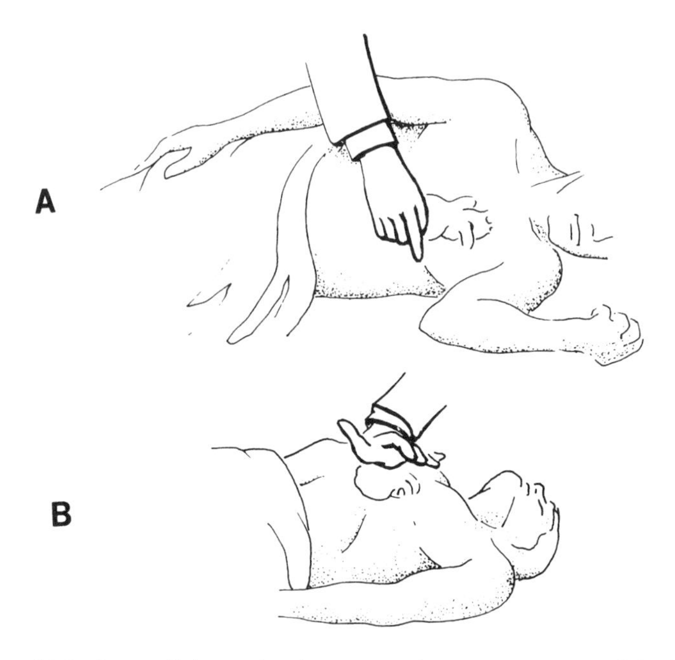

Figure 14-3. Precordial examination in mitral stenosis. (A) Use of the left lateral decubitus recumbent position is mandatory for optimal detection of the murmur of mitral stenosis. The apex impulse is first identified and one finger positioned at this site. The bell of the stethoscope is placed at the apex, using the lightest pressure necessary to make a skin seal. Frequently, the diastolic murmur is audible only over a small precordial area and radiates poorly (see Figure 14-8). (B) Right ventricular activity is felt best with the patient supine and the breath held in mid- or end expiration. Firm pressure with the heel of the hand should be used over the third to fifth interspace at the lower left sternal border. A parasternal lift indicates increased right ventricular hypertrophy or dilatation, possibly augmented by the enlarged left atrium displacing the right ventricle in an anterior direction.

Commonly, an accentuated pulmonic second sound will be palpable in the pulmonic area; its presence in conjunction with a prominent RV lift confirms the diagnosis of pulmonary hypertension.

On occasion, the physical findings in the patient with severe mitral stenosis are those of isolated right heart disease. Evidence for pulmonary hypertension dominates the clinical picture, and mitral valve obstruction may be difficult to diagnose on physical examination. *Practical Point: In adults, severe pulmonary hypertension always is an acquired phenomenon. Mitral stenosis should be considered in such cases, although the classic physical findings may not be present.*

Heart Sounds

First Heart Sound

A loud, snapping S_1 is a hallmark of mitral stenosis. Whenever S_1 is unusually prominent on cardiac examination, evidence of mitral valve disease should be carefully sought.

Amplitude of the S_1 and Opening Snap
There is a direct relationship between audibility and intensity of the first heart sound and opening snap. A loud S_1 and loud OS occur when the mitral leaflets have sufficient mobility and pliability to move rapidly into an open or closed position. When there is calcification, fibrosis, or distortion sufficient to impede leaflet motion, the velocity of leaflet excursion is decreased and the amplitude of S_1 and the opening snap diminish accordingly.

Characteristics of S_1
The first heart sound typically is discrete and loud and has a slapping quality (see Figures 14-2 and 14-4). The increased S_1 is audible throughout the precordium and heard maximally between the lower sternal edge and the apex. The loud S_1 often is palpable.

Opening Snap
An opening snap (OS) is one of the classic findings in cardiac physical diagnosis. *Practical Point: For practical purposes, a loud opening snap indicates a diagnosis of mitral stenosis.* This sound results from the opening of the mitral valve cusps in early diastole. The OS coincides precisely with the maximal opening movement of the anterior leaflet of the mitral valve (see Figures 14-2 and 14-4). On occasion, patients with dominant rheumatic mitral regurgitation will have an OS (see pages 194–195).

Timing (A_2-OS Interval)
The simple *presence* of an OS provides no information as to the severity of the mitral stenosis nor does its intensity have clinical significance except as a marker of leaflet pliability. However, the timing of the OS with respect to S_2 and, specifically, its relationship to the aortic component of S_2 (A_2) may be useful in assessing the severity of the mitral obstruction. The A_2-OS interval has received attention as an indicator

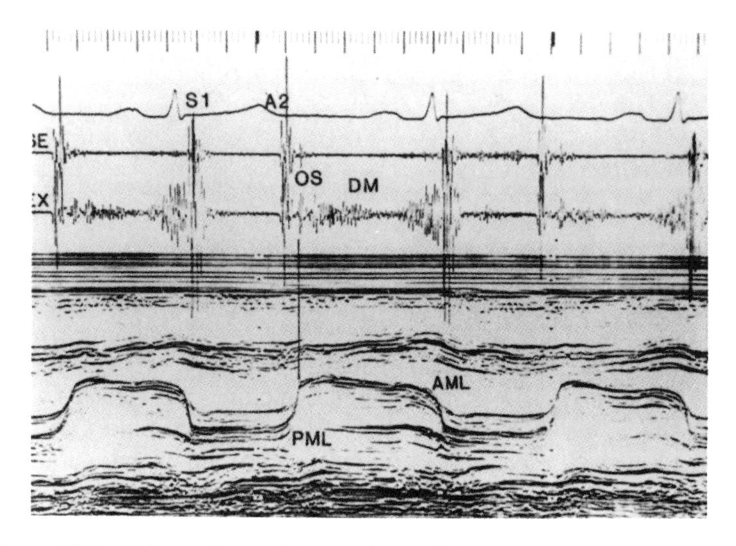

Figure 14-4. Echocardiographic correlates of the loud first sound and opening snap in mitral stenosis. S_1 is produced by mitral valve closure, accentuated and delayed due to elevation of left atrial pressure and the loss of valve compliance. A prominent presystolic diastolic murmur merges with S_1; this represents augmented trasmitral flow with left atrail contraction. The opening snap (OS) times precisely with the maximum opening excursion of the anterior leaflet of the mitral valve, produced by tensing of the valve cusps during early diastole. Left ventricular filling and the resultant early- to mid-diastolic murmur (DM) follows the OS. (Reprinted with permission from Reddy PS, Salerni R, Shaver JA. Normal and abnormal heart sounds in cardiac diagnosis. Part II. Diastolic sounds. *Curr Prog Cardiol.* 1985;10:1.)

of the severity of mitral stenosis. In general a narrow A_2-OS interval indicates severe stenosis, and a long interval suggests mild disease. The timing of these two sounds is related to the level of left atrial pressure. With a high LA pressure, as is found in severe mitral stenosis, the mitral valve opens earlier than normal. In mild to moderate mitral stenosis, LA pressure is less elevated, and the A_2-OS interval therefore is relatively longer. *Practical Point: A short A_2-OS interval (less than 0.08 sec) almost always indicates relatively severe mitral stenosis, although the converse is not true. In some patients, a long A_2-OS interval significantly underestimates the severity of mitral stenosis.*

Acoustic Characteristics
The opening snap typically is a medium- to high-frequency sound, distinct and sharp, that initiates the mitral diastolic rumble. When the OS is of low frequency, it may be confused with an S_3. In general, the OS has an acoustic quality similar to S_1 and S_2. In patients with a mobile anterior leaflet and preserved cardiac output, the OS is prominent and frequently palpable. The OS is heard best inside or medial to the LV apex in the midprecordial area. It may be appreciated best at the left sternal border and, occasionally, is maximal at the cardiac apex. In some patients, the OS is heard better in the left decubitus position.

Aids to Detection
The opening snap should be sought by using firm pressure with the diaphragm of the stethoscope when the subject is in both the supine and left lateral recumbent positions. Mild exercise or handgrip will augment the intensity of the snap.

It may be difficult during auscultation to separate an opening snap from a prominently split S_2, and usually hard to clearly distinguish A_2, P_2, and an OS as three separate sounds during inspiration. Often, the OS is appreciated best or only during expiration. *One must concentrate on detecting all three sound transients by auscultation during many respiratory cycles.*

Optimal auscultation and identification of the OS can be achieved by beginning the inching technique at the pulmonary area and carefully progressing toward the lower left sternal border and apex. Strict attention must be given to the timing and intensity of the various heart sounds during the respiratory cycle at each precordial site of auscultation in both the supine and upright positions.

Decreased Amplitude
One should be alert to conditions or situations where the OS may be quite soft or even absent in the presence of mitral stenosis. The following are conditions frequently associated with a decreased loudness of the opening snap or the first heart sound:

- Severe pulmonary hypertension
- Extensive mitral valve calcification (especially anterior leaflet)
- Congestive heart failure or a very low cardiac output state
- Large right ventricle

- Very mild mitral stenosis
- Mixed mitral valve disease, with dominant mitral regurgitation
- Aortic stenosis (decreased left ventricular compliance)
- Aortic regurgitation

Most important is dense calcification or extensive fibrosis of the mitral valve apparatus or a decreased cardiac output (e.g., congestive heart failure or severe pulmonary hypertension).

Absent Opening Snap

In the presence of dense mitral valve calcification, an opening snap may be present in only one third to one half of subjects. When the right ventricle is dilated, it may occupy the cardiac apex and displace the left ventricle posterolaterally, decreasing the likelihood of detection of the OS.

Differential Diagnosis

Split S_2 A prominent, widely split S_2 may simulate an opening snap, as P_2 is confused for the OS. P_2 is heard best at the pulmonic area without radiation unless there is pulmonary hypertension. The opening snap optimally is detected between the left sternal border (fourth interspace) and the apex and, when loud, can be heard well at the base. A_2-P_2 splitting increases with inspiration; the A_2-OS interval remains constant.

S_3 A third heart sound may be confused for an opening snap. This is particularly true during tachycardia; efforts should be made to slow the heart rate with carotid massage or drug therapy when rapid rates make auscultation difficult. When loud, S_3 often has high-frequency vibrations and more easily is mistaken for an OS. Conversely, the combination of a low- to medium-frequency OS and a long A_2-OS interval can simulate an S_3. The A_2-S_3 interval range (0.10–0.20 sec) is much greater than that of the A_2-OS (0.04–0.14 sec), but there is potential overlap at intervals of 0.10–0.15 sec. During tachycardia, it may be impossible to time these sounds accurately. Compared to the higher-pitched, discrete OS, the S_3 usually is a dull sound of low frequency and low intensity. An S_3 usually is heard only at the apex; it is accentuated in the left lateral decubitus position and softens in the upright position. The OS radiates more widely and is usually equally loud in all positions.

Atrial Myxoma The well-known "tumor plop" of a left atrial myxoma can simulate an opening snap. Usually, it is later, of lower frequency, and more variable in its presence and intensity (Figure 14-5).

Pericardial Knock A loud, medium-high frequency early diastolic sound may be present in constrictive pericarditis. This is the equivalent of an early S_3 and is caused by sudden expansion of the noncompliant left ventricle and pericardium in early diastole. It often produces an audible sound, called a *pericardial knock*, and is easily confused with a mitral OS.

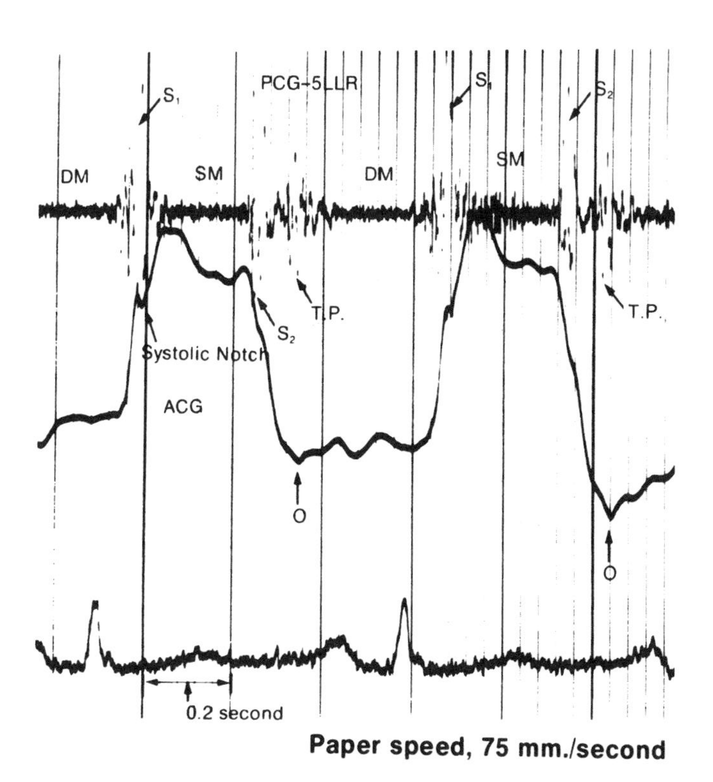

Figure 14-5. Tumor plop of a left atrial myxoma simulating an opening snap. Note the early diastolic sound (TP), which reflects movement of the atrail myxoma toward the left ventricular cavity. Diastolic murmurs (DM) may be produced if the tumor partially obstructs blood flow into the left ventricle. ACG = apex cardiogram. SM = systolic murmur. (Reprinted with permission from Delman AJ, Stein E. *Dynamic Cardiac Auscultation and Phonocardiography*. Philadelphia: WB Saunders Co.; 1979.)

Murmur of Mitral Stenosis

The typical diastolic rumbling murmur of mitral stenosis has two components: an early diastolic murmur that begins with or just after the opening snap and mirrors the rapid filling phase of diastole and a *late* diastolic or presystolic murmur that follows left atrial contraction and represents a sudden accentuation of transvalvular flow just prior to mitral valve closure. In patients with mitral stenosis, either or both murmurs may be heard (see Figures 14-4 and 14-6). The murmur typically begins after the OS, then wanes in intensity, only to increase again at the end of diastole (presystolic accentuation). *Practical Point: It is important to analyze both the early and late portions of diastole for an accurate assessment of the acoustic events in mitral stenosis.*

Early Diastolic Murmur

The first vibrations of the diastolic murmur are coincident with the OS (see Figures 14-2, 14-4, and 14-6). The murmur is loudest in mid-diastole. As flow diminishes in late diastole, the murmur tapers in intensity and may disappear. The presence or absence of the murmur in late diastole depends on the magnitude of the residual left atrial-left ventricular pressure gradient. In severe mitral stenosis or with rapid heart rates, there is a continuous late diastolic gradient and a long diastolic murmur. If the mitral obstruction is only mild to moderate, no gradient or murmur will be present in late diastole. The absence of a late diastolic component is most noticeable following long cycle lengths (Figure 14-7).

Presystolic Murmur

In patients who are in sinus rhythm, late-diastolic enhancement of the earlier-diastolic murmur or an isolated short presystolic murmur occurs following LA systole and the resultant increase in the LA-LV pressure gradient. Thus, the murmur actually crescendos into S_1, producing a presystolic murmur-S_1 complex that may be surprisingly loud (see Figures 14-4 and 14-6).

When atrial fibrillation is present, the presystolic murmur related to LA contraction usually disappears.

Relationship to Severity

Mild Mitral Stenosis

In patients with a small resting LA-LV gradient, there may either be a short, early-diastolic murmur or, on occasion, only a presystolic

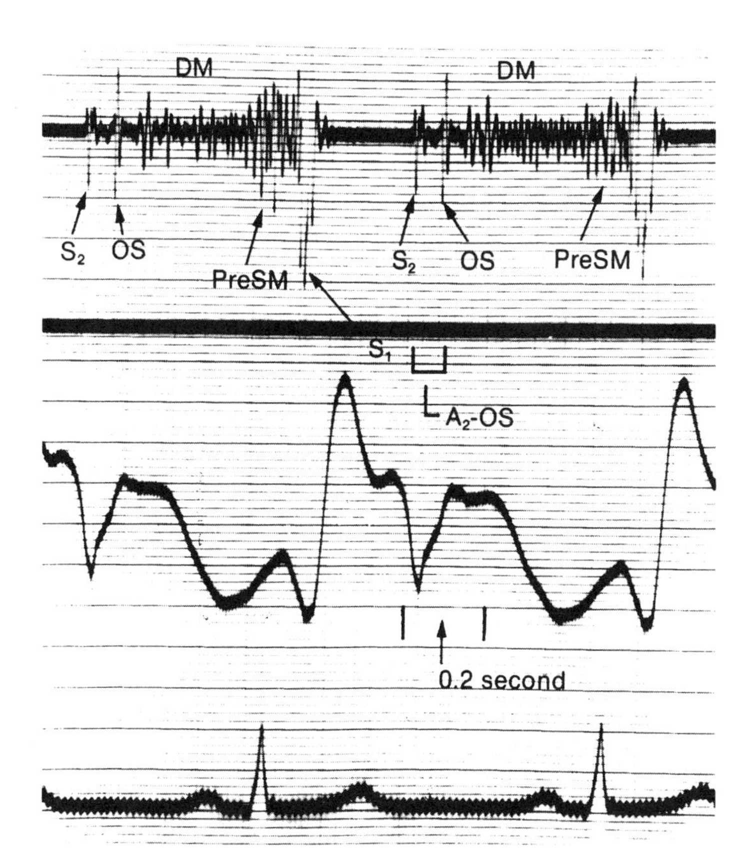

Figure 14-6. Presystolic murmur of mitral stenosis. In this phonocardiogram, the most prominent component of the diastolic murmur is a crescendolike augmentation that follows the left atrail contraction. On auscultation, the presystolic murmur appears to "explode" into a loud S_1. (Reprinted with permission from Delman AJ, Stein E. *Dynamic Cardiac Auscultation and Phonocardiography*. Philadelphia: WB Saunders Co.; 1979.)

crescendo murmur. If both murmurs are present, there usually is a silent gap in mid- to late diastole between the two audible murmur components.

Mild to Moderate Mitral Stenosis

Both the early and late murmurs are heard readily, but a distinct tapering or silence is observed after the middiastolic component.

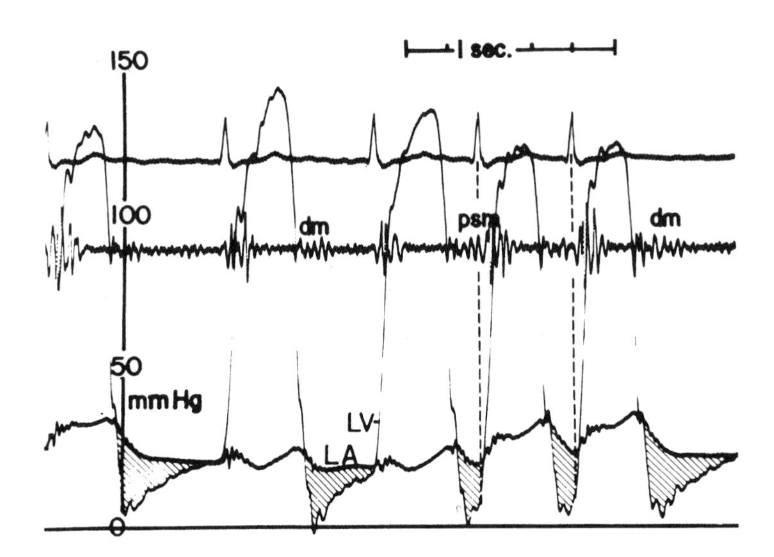

Figure 14-7. Presystolic murmur of mitral stenosis in the presence of atrial fibrillation. Note that, during the short diastolic cycles (third and fourth beats from the left), there is a crescendo presystolic murmur that becomes more accentuated with the onset of left ventricular systole (PSM). During longer cycles, there is an early diastolic murmur but no presystolic component. Thus, a presystolic murmur may be present in the absence of synchronous left atrial contraction. It is produced by a persisting diastolic gradient during short cycles, reflecting continuous diastolic flow across the mitral valve. As the mitral orifice continues to narrow in late diastole, transmitral velocity is augmented and a presystolic murmur immediately precedes S_1. Longer cycle lengths allow adequate time for the left atrium to decompress prior to the onset of left ventricular contraction; mitral valve closure is completed and there is no presystolic murmur. (Reprinted with permission from Criley JM et al. Mitral stenosis: Mechanico-acoustical events. In: Leon DF, Shaver JF, eds. *Physiologic Principles of Heart Sounds and Murmurs*. American Heart Association Monograph No. 46. Armonk, NY: Futura; 1975.)

Moderate to Severe Stenosis

In patients with a substantial and persistent LA-LV gradient, the diastolic rumble truly is *pandiastolic*; sound vibrations start with the opening snap and extend to S_1, typically with an increase in intensity at end diastole (see Figure 14-6). In subjects with slow heart rates or variable cycle lengths during atrial fibrillation, it is important to carefully assess the length of the murmur. *Practical Point: A holodiastolic murmur following the OS during long R-R intervals in sinus rhythm or atrial fibrillation is consistent with major obstruction at the mitral valve level.*

Acoustic Characteristics

Contour

The typical murmur is decrescendo in early diastole and crescendo in late diastole. Long pandiastolic murmurs tend to be even in intensity, with or without presystolic accentuation.

Frequency

The frequency or pitch of the mitral stenosis murmur is low. Analogies between the characteristic rumble of mitral stenosis and distant thunder, the sound of a bowling ball slithering down the alley, or the noise of a distant subway train are fanciful but valid. When mitral flow is relatively rapid, as after mild exercise or in subjects with a good cardiac output, the murmur may be higher pitched. The bell of the stethoscope should be used for auscultation of all but the very loudest murmurs of mitral stenosis. *Use only the lightest pressure necessary to make a skin seal. Practical Point: The left recumbent position is mandatory to enhance detection of the low-frequency vibrations that become much more audible with this maneuver* (see Figures 14-3A and 14-8). Often the diastolic rumble can be heard only with the patient in the left decubitus position.

Location

One of the difficulties in detection of the murmur of mitral stenosis is the limited precordial area over which the murmur is heard. With murmurs of low to medium intensity, the zone of auscultation often is small and localized to the apex impulse in the left recumbent position. The murmur may be inaudible in the supine position. *Practical Point: Careful identification of the apical impulse with one finger and simultaneous application of the bell of the stethoscope in the left lateral position is mandatory for auscultation of the mitral stenosis murmur in many patients* (see Figure 14-3A). The murmur may be inaudible even 1–2 cm away from this area.

Radiation

The low-intensity mitral stenosis murmur is well localized and usually does not radiate appreciably. When the murmur is of medium frequency and medially located, it can simulate the diastolic murmur of aortic regurgitation.

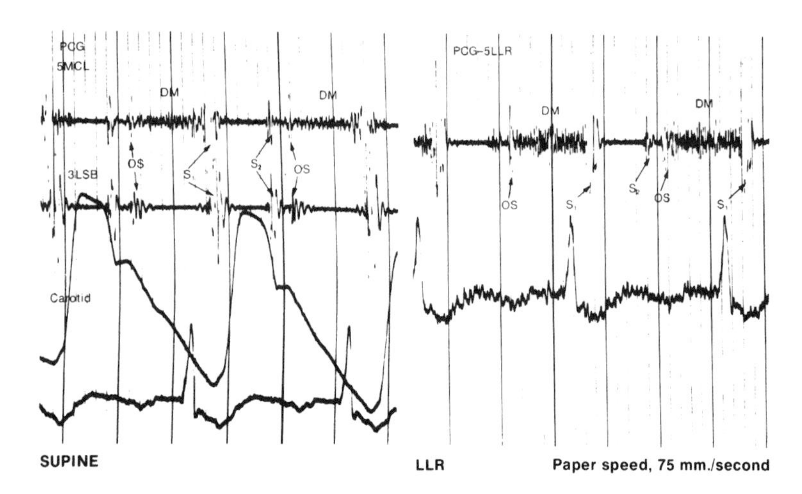

Figure 14-8. Augmentation of the diastolic murmur of mitral stenosis in the left lateral position. This sequence of phonocardiograms demonstrates the increase in the intensity of the diastolic murmur that occurs when the patient is turned to the left lateral position. The gain settings of the phonocardiogram are the same. DM = diastolic murmur; OS = opening snap. (Reprinted with permission from Delman AJ, Stein E. *Dynamic Cardiac Auscultation and Phonocardiography*. Philadelphia: WB Saunders Co.; 1979.)

Intensity

The loudness of the mitral rumble does not bear as consistent a relationship to the severity of the obstruction as the length of the murmur. The intensity of the murmur of mitral stenosis is related directly to the velocity of blood flow across the mitral valve and the severity of the stenosis. High flows result in loud murmurs; a narrow valve orifice produces an increased velocity of blood flow if the stroke volume is maintained. However, when mitral stenosis becomes severe, flow velocity may diminish as the stroke volume falls. Mitral stenosis murmurs may be so loud as to produce an apical thrill in the left decubitus position, particularly in thin patients. Many subjects with mitral stenosis have a murmur of such softness as to make detection difficult. This is discussed in the section "Aids to Detection of Mitral Stenosis." Table 14-1 lists the causes of the decreased murmur intensity of mitral stenosis.

Silent Mitral Stenosis

It is uncommon for mitral stenosis to be truly undetectable or silent, but this situation does occur. In very mild mitral stenosis with a large

Table 14-1. Factors Associated with Decreased Intensity of the Diastolic Rumble of Mitral Stenosis

- Low flow states
  - Severe mitral stenosis
  - Severe pulmonary hypertension
  - Congestive heart failure
  - Atrial fibrillation, especially with rapid ventricular rate
- Characteristics of the mitral valve
  - Extensive calcification of the mitral apparatus
  - Subvalvular chordal obliteration
  - Left atrial thrombus protruding into mitral orifice
  - Anatomic distortion of the mitral valve with posteromedial deviation of the orifice
- Associated cardiac lesions
  - Aortic stenosis
  - Aortic regurgitation
  - Atrial septal defect
  - Pulmonary hypertension with marked RV enlargement
- Other
  - Cardiac apex formed by right ventricle
  - Inability to localize cardiac apex, due to
    - Obesity
    - COPD
    - Muscular chest
    - Large breasts

mitral valve orifice and a small gradient, the murmur may be absent. The most common cause of silent mitral stenosis is poor auscultatory technique, such as improper application of the stethoscope (failure to use the left decubitus position, failure to use light pressure with the bell), erroneous identification of the cardiac apex, lack of the use of murmur enhancement techniques (see later), or misinterpretation of the cardiac findings. Nevertheless, mitral stenosis truly can be inaudible when there is low blood flow regardless of the cause. With RV dilatation, the apex impulse may not be left ventricular in origin and is occupied by the right ventricle. In such cases, the murmur may be audible only in the left or midaxillary line and should be carefully sought in this area. Very severe mitral stenosis, associated pulmonary hypertension and combination lesions (e.g., aortic valve disease) commonly result in silent mitral stenosis on auscultation.

Factors Increasing the Intensity
In combined mitral regurgitation and stenosis, an increased volume of left atrial blood accentuates both the intensity and duration of the mitral rumble. In general, males tend to have louder murmurs than females. Tachycardia or short cycle lengths during atrial fibrillation also increase murmur intensity.

Aids to Detection of Mitral Stenosis

The proper use of the stethoscope (light pressure with bell at the cardiac apex in the left decubitus position) has been emphasized. Auscultation should be performed in mid- or end expiration; the faint mitral rumble easily can be masked by respiratory sounds. It is surprising how easily the rumble is heard when the patient is auscultated in the process of turning onto the left side or immediately after assuming the left recumbent position (see Figure 14-8); this probably is related to a brief increase in heart rate and transvalvular flow occurring during the turning maneuver. *Practical Point: Anything that increases the heart rate and/or the left atrial–left ventricular gradient enhances audibility of the mitral rumble.* The most practical maneuvers to accomplish this include (1) asking the patient to cough deeply several times in succession; (2) using mild exercise, such as sit-ups or deep knee bends; or (3) listening while the patient changes from the squatting to the supine or left lateral position. Isometric effort in the form of a sustained handgrip also may be useful. Some advocate having the patient breathe deeply several times in rapid succession to accelerate the heart rate.

Identification of Systole and Diastole

Diastole easily is confused with systole in patients with mitral stenosis, particularly when there are no other associated murmurs and the heart rate is relatively fast. A prominent opening snap can be readily mistaken for S_1, with the diastolic murmur appearing to be systolic in timing. The loud S_1 is confused for S_2 (Figure 14-9). Rapid heart rates and atrial fibrillation accentuate this problem.

Practical Point: Always utilize careful simultaneous palpation of the carotid artery or apex impulse to accurately identify S_1 and S_2 and define the OS and the proper sequence of systole and diastole. The "inching technique" is helpful in preventing this confusion; S_1 and S_2 are identified more easily at the base, where the OS may be heard but the diastolic murmur will be absent. Careful inching of the stethoscope toward the apex after definite identification of these cardiac sounds will avoid confusing systole with diastole.

Differential Diagnosis

A number of conditions can simulate mitral stenosis. Any cause of enhanced A-V valve flow may result in an S_3 and short middiastolic murmur, a sound complex mistaken for an opening snap and mitral stenosis rumble.

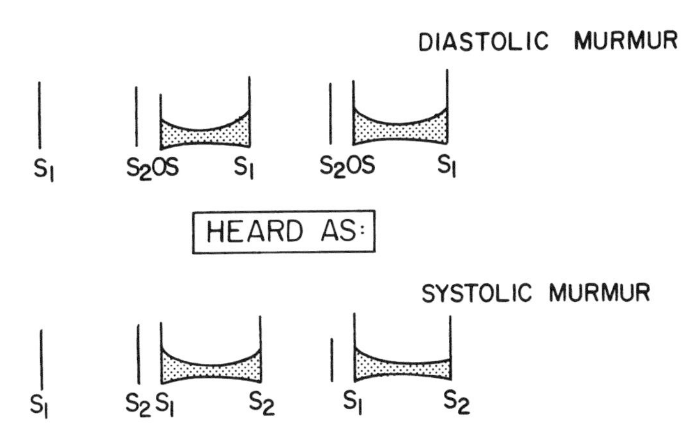

Figure 14-9. Auscultatory confusion of diastole for systole in mitral stenosis. This diagram indicates how an observer can mistake the diastolic murmur of mitral stenosis for a systolic murmur. The opening snap is heard readily as an "S_1" and systole is confused with diastole. Because physicians are used to hearing the majority of murmurs in systole, the acoustic findings in pure mitral stenosis can be misleading. This is particularly true if the underlying heart rate is rapid. Careful attention to the proper identification of S_1 and S_2 is essential to the correct interpretation of cardiac events.

Conditions associated with prominent diastolic filling sounds and murmurs simulating mitral stenosis include

- Thyrotoxicosis
- Atrial septal defect
- Anemia
- Ventricular septal defect
- Third-degree A-V block
- Patent ductus arteriosus
- Mitral regurgitation (pure)
- Ebstein's anomaly
- Large left ventricle (cardiomyopathy)
- Severe aortic regurgitation (Austin Flint murmur)

Tricuspid Stenosis

Patients with rheumatic tricuspid stenosis have a tricuspid opening snap and diastolic rumble on examination. Inspiratory augmentation of the diastolic murmur and maximal intensity at the lower sternal border favor tricuspid stenosis. The jugular A wave should be prominent (in the absence of atrial fibrillation).

Left Atrial Myxoma

Obstruction of the mitral valve orifice by tumor can simulate mitral stenosis. The resultant murmur often is solely presystolic. S_1 may be increased and an opening snap may be present (tumor plop, see Figure 14-5). The acoustic findings may vary from day to day. Echocardiography has caused embarrassment to many clinicians who previously diagnosed mitral stenosis when, subsequently, the patient was found to have a left atrial myxoma.

Constrictive Pericarditis

The early, loud pericardial knock can mimic an opening snap. However, S_1 typically is not increased and a diastolic murmur is not present. The jugular venous pulse manifests prominent X and Y troughs and invariably has an elevated mean pressure.

Austin Flint Murmur

An apical rumbling murmur in the presence of aortic regurgitation represents mitral stenosis or an Austin Flint murmur. This differential diagnosis is discussed in Chapter 12. The lack of a loud S_1 and an opening snap are the most valuable criteria for exclusion of the diagnosis of mitral stenosis in patients with aortic regurgitation. The combination of rheumatic aortic regurgitation and mitral stenosis is common. However, the true Austin Flint murmur is found only with severe aortic regurgitation.

15

Mitral Valve Prolapse

Mitral valve prolapse (MVP) is a relatively common abnormality of the mitral valve. The spectrum of MVP ranges from an isolated systolic click in an asymptomatic individual to full-blown, severe mitral regurgitation necessitating mitral valve replacement (floppy valve syndrome). Many cases are discovered accidentally during routine physical examination. Affected individuals may have a variety of symptoms such as palpitations, atypical chest pain, or dyspnea. Anxiety, fatigue, and occasionally syncope also may occur in symptomatic patients. It remains uncertain if these symptoms truly are related to MVP. Rare sudden deaths have been reported, presumably caused by malignant ventricular dysrhythmias.

MVP has a multitude of names and eponyms. The term *mitral valve prolapse* is most desirable, although many authors still refer to MVP as *Barlow's syndrome.*

A spectrum of noncardiac abnormalities has been associated with the mitral valve prolapse syndrome. These include evidence for a hyperadrenergic state as well as enhanced vagal activity. Some individuals with MVP have been shown to have a variety of arrhythmias.

Pathophysiology

The basic defect of MVP is an alteration in the composition of the mitral valve tissue and chordae. The normal dense collagen fibers (fibrosa) are lost or destroyed and replaced and invaded by a less sturdy type of connective tissue (spongiosa) that has increased amounts of uronic acid mucopolysaccharide material. The resultant myxomatous transformation may affect individual scallops or an entire mitral cusp. One or both leaflets may be involved. The chordae tendineae also may be abnormal, often elongated and attenuated. The mitral leaflet tissue itself often is thickened, redundant, and excessive (Figure 15-1). During systole individual scallops or an entire leaflet billow excessively into the left atrium.

Criley aptly depicted the mitral valve in MVP as being being "too big" for the left ventricle; the valve leaflets protrude or prolapse abnormally above the mitral annulus during ventricular contraction. Mitral regurgitation, if present, occurs when loss of normal coaptation results from true prolapse of the mitral leaflet due to either protrusion of the redundant valve tissue or abnormally long and lax chordae.

Mitral regurgitation, when present, typically is confined to *late systole* and occurs as the size of the left ventricular chamber has decreased maximally and the anatomic extent of prolapse is greatest. In subjects with severe prolapse, the murmur and the mitral regurgitation may be holosystolic.

Both mitral leaflets can be affected in MVP, but more commonly the posterior (mural) cusp is involved. The posterior leaflet has a greater potential for prolapse, probably because of its multiple scallops and less adequate chordal support than in the anterior cusp. For severe mitral regurgitation to be present, both leaflets must be affected or one cusp may be flail, as with a ruptured chordae tendineae. In such individuals, the mitral valve tissue is predictably voluminous and eccentrically thickened. In severe mitral valve prolapse, the mitral valve annulus often is quite dilated.

Etiology

Many conditions have been associated with mitral valve prolapse (Table 15-1). It is best to categorize prolapse as either a *primary* or *secondary* disorder. By far the most common, primary cases represent

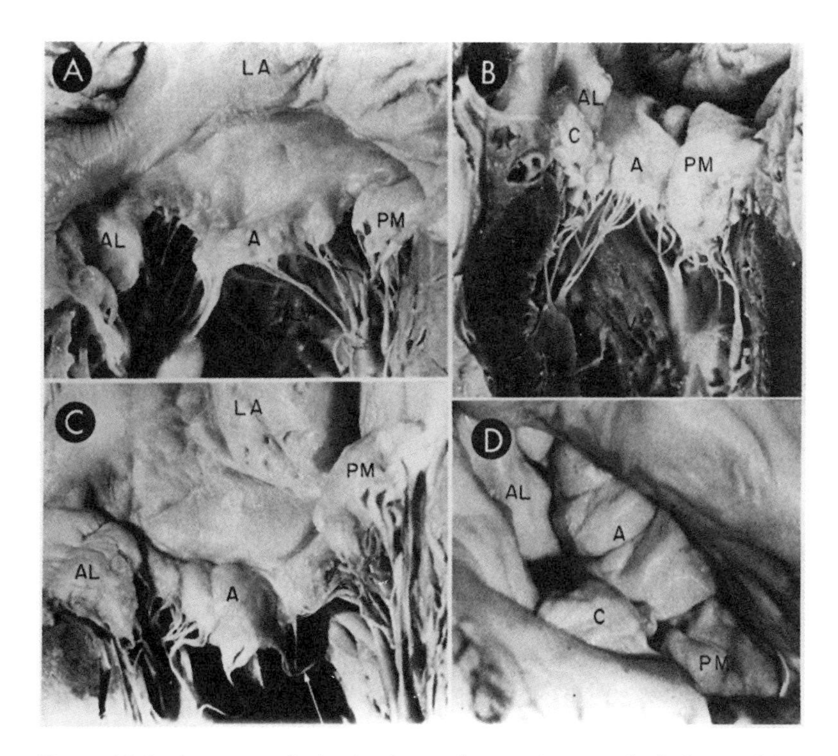

Figure 15-1. Anatomy of mitral valve prolapse. (A) Note the bulging of the outer portion of the anterior leaflet and hooding of the posteromedial and anterolateral scallops of the posterior leaflet. (B) Here, the degree of prolapse is more advanced, with hooding of the anterior leaflet as well as hooding of all three scallops of the posterior leaflet. (C) Note the hooding of the anterior leaflet, the posteromedial, and anterolateral scallops. Two ruptured chordae are attached to the anterior leaflet, with elongated and thinned chordae elsewhere. (D) This is the same specimen as in B, with the mitral valve viewed from the atrium. AL = anterolateral scallop; PM = posteromedial scallop; C = central scallop; A = anterior leaflet; LA = left atrium. (Reprinted with permission from Lucas RV, Edwards JE. The floppy mitral valve. *Curr Probl Cardiol.* 1982;7:1.)

an idiopathic abnormality of mitral valve tissue that appears to have its onset after childhood. MVP is uncommon in children.

Primary mitral valve prolapse is familial, transmitted as an autosomal dominant trait with incomplete penetrance. The rare systemic connective tissue disorders such as Marfan syndrome, Erdheim's cystic medial necrosis, von Willebrand's syndrome, and Ehlers-Danlos

Table 15-1. Conditions Associated with Mitral Valve Prolapse

Floppy valve syndrome (myxomatous degeneration)
Marfan syndrome
Ehlers-Danlos syndrome
Willebrand syndrome
Atrial septal defect
Rheumatic mitral valve disease
Hypertrophic cardiomyopathy
Hyperthyroidism
Straight back syndrome
Muscular dystrophy
Wolff-Parkinson-White syndrome
Lupus erythematosus
Relapsing polychondritis
Pseudoxanthoma elasticum

syndrome have an extremely high incidence of mitral valve prolapse, but primary or idiopathic mitral prolapse is unrelated to these unusual conditions in most affected individuals.

Patients with secondum atrial septal defects and hypertrophic cardiomyopathy appear to have an increased prevalence of MVP on echocardiography, particularly patients with atrial septal defect.

A number of serious complications may occur in patients with MVP (Table 15-2). It remains a subject of controversy as to whether these clinical events are truly causally related to MVP. Therefore, it is of more than academic importance to accurately detect this condition on physical examination. For instance, this diagnosis suggests a need for antibiotic prophylaxis to prevent bacterial endocarditis. MVP is a clinical entity best delineated by auscultation and echocardiography. In the absence of a click or late systolic murmur on repeated examination, an individual should not be labeled as having the MVP syndrome solely from echocardiographic findings. Patients with prolapse on echocardiography who are asymptomatic or have symptoms of atypical chest pain or palpations but a consistently normal cardiac examination fall into a most difficult diagnostic category. Some clinicians consider these subjects to have true MVP, but others do not.

Table 15-2. Serious Complications of Mitral Valve Prolapse

Bacterial endocarditis
Transient cerebral ischemic attacks
Cerebral (or systemic) emboli
Severe mitral regurgitation (floppy mitral valve syndrome)
Congestive heart failure
Necessity for mitral valve replacement
Sudden death (rare)

Physical Examination

General Appearance

Mitral valve prolapse is one of the few cardiac conditions in adults where the outward appearance of the subject may suggest the diagnosis. Individuals with the familial variety of prolapse often are red haired and fair skinned. Affected subjects have an increased prevalence of nonspecific skeletal abnormalities in both the nonfamilial and familial varieties. Many patients are thin or asthenic, with long extremities. Some degree of pectus excavatum and, less commonly, pectus carinatum is common. Scoliosis and loss of the normal dorsal thoracic kyphosis frequently is observed; a narrow A-P chest diameter (straight back) may be present. Recently, MVP has been associated with very small breasts in women (hypomastia).

The incidence of such minor skeletal abnormalities in perhaps 20–30% of patients with primary mitral valve prolapse suggests an embryonic defect in mesenchymal formation that has been called a *linked mesenchymal dysplasia.* Formation of the atrioventricular valves, mitral annulus, and atrial septum secundum, as well as chondrification and ossification of the skeletal cage, all occur around the sixth to seventh week of gestation. Breast differentiation begins at this time. Therefore, a common but unidentified embryologic defect of connective tissue formation or structure may be a link to our ultimate understanding of mitral valve prolapse.

Carotid and Jugular Venous Pulse

No detectable abnormalities of the arterial or venous pulse are present in most individuals with mitral prolapse.

Precordial Motion

The apex impulse in MVP is normal on palpation. Because associated mitral regurgitation, when present, typically is mild, the left ventricle does not enlarge. When severe mitral regurgitation is present, the apical impulse is hyperdynamic and may be displaced leftward if there is LV dilatation (see Chapters 4 and 13 and Figure 13-3).

Heart Sounds

Patients with MVP have no predictable abnormalities of the first and second heart sounds. S_1 usually is normal in intensity. In the unusual case of a flail mitral leaflet and gross mitral regurgitation, S_1 may be attenuated or even absent. An increase in intensity of S_1 may occur if the click is close to or coincides with S_1.

When present, the degree of mitral reflux in MVP usually is only mild to moderate; therefore, the widely split S_2 common to severe mitral regurgitation is not found in most patients with prolapse.

The Click(s)

Practical Point: The presence of a single click or multiple systolic clicks in mild to late systole is the most specific auscultatory feature of mitral valve prolapse (Figure 15-2). The clicks in MVP are brief, high-frequency, popping or snapping sounds produced by the systolic billowing of the mitral valve leaflets or individual scallops and are synchronous with the maximal prolapsing motion of the involved valve tissue. When multiple clicks are present, one click usually is more prominent than others (see Figure 15-2). The clicks often are variable in timing and may change their position within systole (see later). Multiple clicks frequently are present but often missed by the inexperienced examiner. A series of high-frequency clicks typically sounds like a faint crackling or rustling noise. The clicks often appear to be disassociated from the murmur and may have a metallic quality. When several clicks are present in succession, the resultant sound may be mistaken for a scratchy systolic murmur.

MVP clicks typically appear to be "close to the ear." It is important to concentrate or tune in to the high-frequency range to best detect midsystolic clicks; having the patient hold his or her breath is helpful for optimal auscultation. Clicks often are very faint. Acoustically, they are dissimilar to the far more common low-frequency cardiac sounds (e.g., S_3 or S_4). The clicks (as well as the murmur) may vary in intensity and number over time and be present inconsistently, even on a beat-to-beat basis. A prominent systolic murmur easily can obscure the presence of clicks unless the examiner concentrates on different frequency ranges during auscultation. *Practical Point: Many patients with mitral valve prolapse have only a midsystolic click or multiple clicks with no late or holosystolic murmur. The absence of a murmur indicates the absence of mitral regurgitation.*

Timing of the Click

The midsystolic click of mitral valve prolapse, in contradistinction to an ejection click, bears no relationship to ejection of blood from the heart. The clicks coincide with the precise moment of prolapse of the leaflet or a scallop, which usually occurs after left ventricular systolic size has decreased considerably. Therefore, the click normally is found

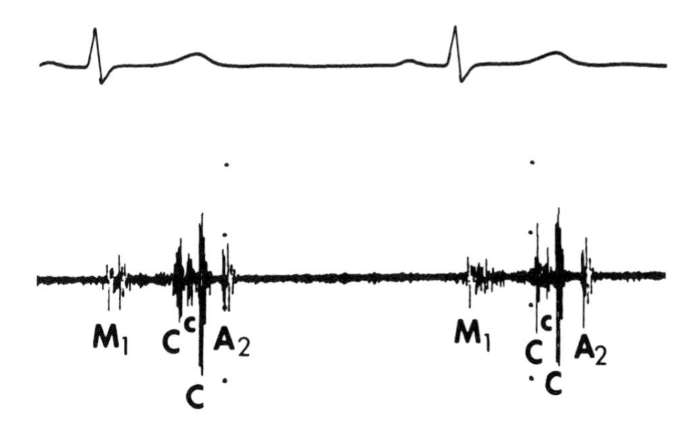

Figure 15-2. Multiple systolic clicks in a patient with mitral valve prolapse. There are at least three dominant clicks, with the loudest in late systole. (Reprinted with permission from Cheitlin MD, Byrd RC. Prolapsed mitral valve: The commonest valve disease? *Curr Probl Cardiol.* 1984;8:1.)

in *mid- to late systole*, not during early systole (Figure 15-3A). Nevertheless, the click of MVP may occur just after S_1 (Figure 15-3B) or be simultaneous with S_1 when the onset of the prolapse occurs very early in systole (Figure 15-3C). Obviously, in the latter case, it is extremely difficult to diagnose a click except with multiple examinations using a variety of patient positions and during various maneuvers.

An early click may simulate a loud S_1, a split S_1, or an S_1-ejection sound complex (Figures 15-3 and 15-4). When very early prolapse occurs, the click can move into S_1 and a separate sound may not be audible; S_1 appears to be increased in intensity (see Figure 15-3C). Whenever one hears a loud "S_1" in conjunction with a holosystolic murmur, it should suggest the diagnosis of holosystolic mitral leaflet prolapse.

Alterations in the timing of a nonejection click with pharmacologic agents or other maneuvers correlate closely with the behavior of the systolic murmur (Table 15-3). Therefore, the click moves closer to S_1 when the subject assumes the upright posture; the systolic murmur lengthens and the murmur vibrations extend toward S_1. Squatting decreases the duration and extent of mitral prolapse by increasing left ventricular volume; both the click and murmur are heard later in systole.

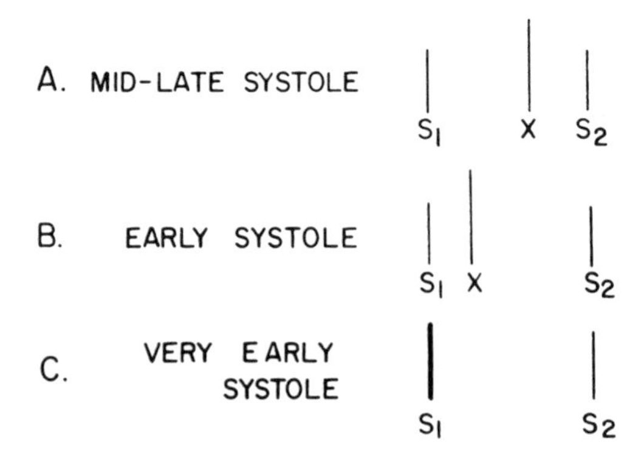

Figure 15-3. Variable timing of the systolic click in mitral valve prolapse. While the click (X) typically is heard in mid- to late systole (A), it may be head in early systole if prolapse of one or more leaflets begins shortly after ejection (B). In holosystolic prolapse, the first heart sound often is accentuated, suggesting superimposition of the click on the normal S_1 (C).

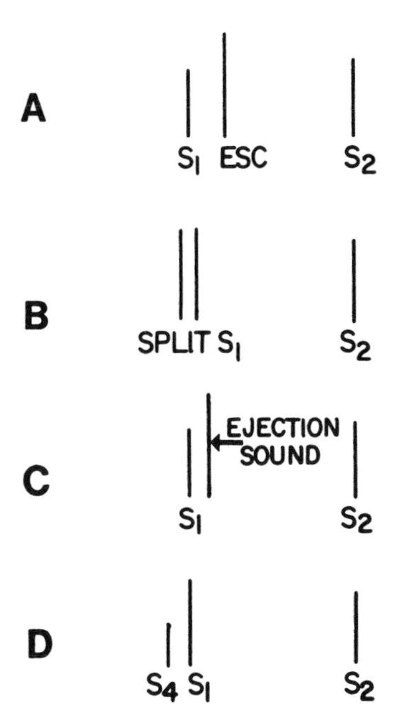

Figure 15-4. Differential diagnosis of an early systolic click (see the text). ESC = click.

The Isolated Click

The diagnosis of MVP should be suspected strongly whenever a midsystolic click is heard. Many asymptomatic subjects demonstrate a click or several clicks only and no murmur at all (see Figure 15-2). The murmur may vary in its presence from day to day.

Optimal Auscultation of Systolic Clicks

Because clicks often are difficult to detect, one should be prepared to bring out these sounds during auscultation. Firm pressure with the stethoscope diaphragm is optimal for detection of these high-pitched, brief-snapping sounds. Clicks usually are heard best at the apex or more medially toward the lower sternum.

The maneuvers used to enhance detection of mitral valve prolapse are discussed later. Careful auscultation with the patient in the supine, left recumbent, and sitting or standing positions is important for optimal detection of the click and any accompanying murmur.

Table 15-3. Characteristic Variations with Different Maneuvers of Click and Murmur Produced by Mitral Valve Prolapse

Intervention	Resultant Functional Change	Acoustic Consequences
Upright posture, sitting or standing	Decrease LV volume, earlier prolapse	C moves closer to S_1, often louder LSM becomes longer, may become holosystolic: Peaks earlier in systole M may become louder
Long cycle lengths (post-PVC beats, during atrial fibrillation, bradycardia)	Larger LV volume, later prolapse	No change or decrease in M intensity, shorter M, later C
Left decubitus position	Heart closer to stethoscope	C and M may be louder
Inspiration	Decrease LVEDV, increase HR	C and M move toward S_1 M unchanged or louder; may decrease in intensity C variably decreased in intensity
Valsalva maneuver		
Strain	Decrease LVEDV, increase heart rate	C earlier, softer M may transiently decrease in early phase (first 30 sec) M earlier, often louder later during strain M can become holosystolic, musical
Release	Increase LVEDV, bradycardia	Increase intensity of M and C to baseline by 6–8 beats after release M and C can occur later (if overshoot)

Isometric handgrip	Increase systemic vascular resistance, increase BP	Increase intensity of C and M C and M may occur earlier in systole
Squatting	Increase systemic vascular resistance Increase abdominal pressure Increase venous return Increase systolic BP Increase LVEDV Reflex bradycardia	Delay in onset of C and M (prolapse may disappear) Decrease M intensity; variable M response
Amyl nitrite	Decrease LVEDV, increase heart rate	C and M move toward S_1, LSM may appear or become holosystolic C and M may become louder

M = murmur; C = click; LSM = late systolic murmur; EDV = end-diastolic volume; HR = heart rate; BP = blood pressure; LV = left ventricular.

Differential Diagnosis of the Midsystolic Click

A mid- or late-systolic click readily can be mistaken for part of a widely split S_2 complex if the click is assumed to be A_2. An opening snap is another acoustic event simulated by mitral prolapse. In this case, the click is mistaken for S_2, and the actual S_2 is believed to be the opening snap. The presence of a late systolic murmur can add to this acoustic problem, as it may be easily mistaken for an early diastolic murmur if the click is confused for S_2 (Figure 15-5).

Murmur of Mitral Valve Prolapse

Characteristically, the murmur of mitral valve prolapse begins in mid- to late systole (Figure 15-6). It typically fans out to S_2, like all murmurs of late mitral regurgitation. The prolapse murmur sounds like the systolic murmur of papillary muscle dysfunction and, in fact, may be acoustically indistinguishable if there is no associated systolic click. Perhaps 30–40% of identified subjects with mitral valve prolapse

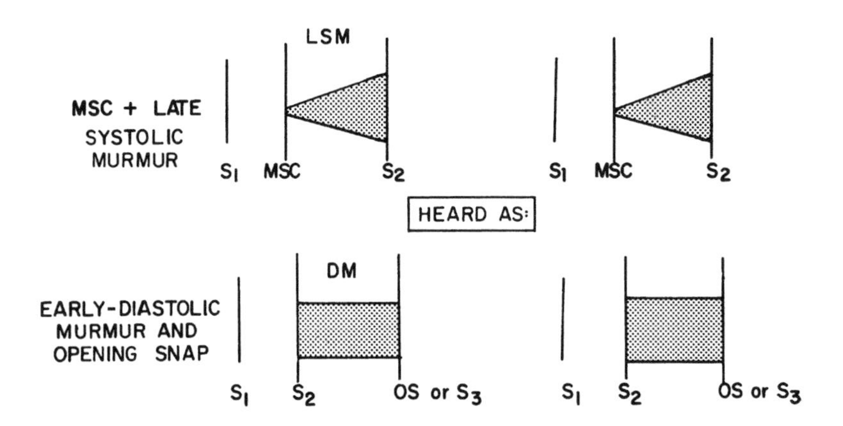

Figure 15-5. Confusion of the midsystolic click–late-systolic murmur for a diastolic murmur and opening snap. Because physicians are used to hearing the majority of murmurs in early to midsystole, a late-systolic murmur frequently is confused for a diastolic murmur, particularly when it follows a prominent click that is mistaken for S_2. It is not uncommon for patients with classic findings of the click-murmur syndrome to receive a diagnosis of mitral stenosis.

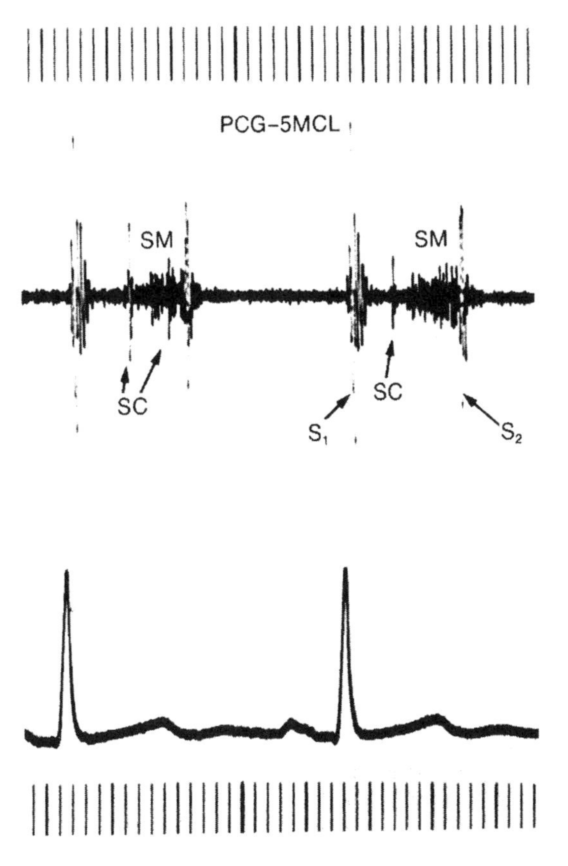

Figure 15-6. The classic late systolic murmur of mitral valve prolapse. Note the crescendo configuration of the murmur, which begins in midsystole following the first systolic click. The frequency of this murmur usually is relatively pure. SM = systolic murmur. SC = systolic click. (Reprinted with permission from Delman AJ, Stein E. *Dynamic Cardiac Auscultation and Phonocardiography*. Philadelphia: WB Saunders Co.; 1979.)

have both a click and a murmur. A majority have a click only, and a minority have only a late systolic murmur. Definite MVP has been documented by M-mode or two-dimensional echocardiography or left ventricular angiography in individuals *with no auscultatory* clues for MVP; that is, no murmur and no click. It is unclear whether these "silent" cases of prolapse fit into the broader MVP syndrome.

Intensity

Because the degree of mitral regurgitation, when present, usually is mild, the systolic murmur typically is soft. However, the late systolic component occasionally displays considerable accentuation and may be prominent. If a systolic whoop or honk is present (see later), these auscultatory phenomena can be very loud indeed. Various maneuvers can accentuate or diminish the amplitude of the murmur. *Practical Point: The intensity of the MVP murmur is extremely variable. In some persons, the murmur may be inaudible in one position but grade 2–4/6 intensity in another position. The murmur also may vary several grades with various maneuvers.*

Frequency

Murmurs of MVP usually are medium to high pitched. They typically are of relatively pure frequency and have a whirring or regurgitant quality.

Timing

The mid- to late-systolic nature of the murmur of mitral prolapse is characteristic, despite considerable variability in the timing of murmur onset related to different body positions and various physical maneuvers.

A prolapse murmur that begins in early systole or clearly is holosystolic suggests moderate to severe mitral regurgitation and indicates that the abnormal prolapsing leaflet motion begins with or near the onset of ejection. A pansystolic murmur of MVP occurs in approximately 10% of the subjects with MVP. In these patients, significant mitral regurgitation may result in left atrial and left ventricular enlargement. The term *floppy valve syndrome* has been applied loosely to such patients with MVP and major mitral regurgitation. Associated midsystolic clicks are not likely to be present in such individuals, although an increased S_1 intensity is common. The diagnosis of a floppy mitral valve related to the myxomatous leaflet changes characteristic of primary MVP is made best by echocardiography or during left ventricular angiography or an operation. This condition is the most common cause of severe chronic mitral regurgitation in adults.

Contour

The murmur of MVP typically is crescendo in late systole (see Figure 15-6). Early-systolic murmurs that taper in late systole (ejection quality) usually do not represent MVP. A pansystolic murmur, with or without associated clicks, can be caused by holosystolic prolapse. If a pansystolic murmur has a late systolic accentuation, the underlying etiologic possibilities also include papillary muscle dysfunction, a calcified mitral annulus, or rheumatic mitral regurgitation.

Systolic Whoops and Honks

Occasionally, patients with mitral valve prolapse develop peculiar loud vibratory or musical systolic murmurs, known as *whoops* or *honks*. Usually, these come and go in an intermittent fashion and may appear and disappear suddenly during auscultation. They often are initiated by changes in body position such as standing or sitting forward. Typically, the patient has the classic acoustic findings of midsystolic MVP, which abruptly become more pronounced, initiating a whoop. These murmurs can be so loud that the patient may hear them.

Effects of Body Position, Drugs, and Physical Maneuvers

The use of ancillary maneuvers (see Table 15-3) and pharmacologic agents in auscultation is most rewarding in several cardiac conditions, such as hypertrophic cardiomyopathy and mitral valve prolapse. The murmurs of both disorders behave in a similar fashion with *most* but *not all* interventions: In both conditions, the underlying pathophysiologic abnormality is accentuated by any alteration that produces a *smaller left ventricular cavity* or an *increase in the force of contraction*. In MVP, such maneuvers cause the prolapse to occur earlier in systole, moving the click(s) and murmur closer to S_1 and increasing the duration of the mitral regurgitation, if present. The opposite occurs when left ventricular cavity size abruptly increases. Alterations in left ventricular preload and afterload also produce predictable changes in the timing of the onset of the click and murmur.

Table 15-3 summarizes the typical responses of the click and murmur to a variety of altered physiologic states and body positions. *Practical Point: The behavior of the timing of the click and murmur is of greater diagnostic usefulness than changes in intensity.* Often the acoustic abnormalities may be minimal or even absent at rest in the supine position but obvious when the patient is upright or turned onto the left side. *Practical Point: In any patient suspected of or known to have MVP, auscultation should be carried out with the subject in the supine, left lateral, sitting forward, and standing positions. It also may be helpful to listen while the subject squats and then abruptly returns to the standing position.*

Differential Diagnosis

For the experienced clinician, the classic finding of a prominent non-ejection click and a late systolic murmur should not be confused for other cardiovascular abnormalities. Holosystolic murmurs must be differentiated from other causes of mitral regurgitation, such as rheumatic heart disease; the diagnosis of MVP in such cases is suggested if there is a prominent click (rare) or a loud S_1, but the etiology must be confirmed by an echocardiogram. *Hypertrophic cardiomyopathy* may be confused with mitral valve prolapse in patients who have only a mid- to late-systolic murmur; an LV heave presence of an S_4, the absence of a click, and exaggeration of the murmur following a PVC strongly favor hypertrophic cardiomyopathy. The murmur in this condition usually has prominent ejection characteristics (see Chapter 11).

The late systolic murmur of *papillary muscle dysfunction* typically is accompanied by an S_3 or S_4, along with some evidence of left ventricular dysfunction (see Figure 13-9). Papillary muscle murmurs do not increase in the upright posture. A midsystolic click is not heard. However, auscultatory evidence of MVP has been documented in patients with coronary artery disease following myocardial infarction. Therefore, a late systolic murmur that fans out to S_2 can be a manifestation of either MVP or papillary muscle dysfunction. Patients with *coarctation of the aorta* may have a late systolic murmur and an early (ejection) click. The maximal intensity of the murmur away from the cardiac apex (high left chest and interscapular) excludes MVP.

16

Tricuspid Regurgitation

Tricuspid regurgitation usually is not viewed as an important valve lesion; yet this abnormality is far more common than generally appreciated. A common denominator of tricuspid regurgitation in adults is the presence of pulmonary hypertension. Signs of elevated pulmonary artery pressure (increased P_2, right ventricular lift) always should stimulate a careful search for tricuspid regurgitation; conversely, any suggestion of tricuspid regurgitation on clinical examination should provoke a meticulous evaluation for evidence of an increased pulmonary artery pressure.

Functional Anatomy

The tricuspid valve consists of a septal leaflet, an anterior leaflet, and a posterior leaflet, each anchored via the chordae tendineae. The anterior cusp is the most mobile leaflet.

As with the mitral valve it is useful to think of a *tricuspid valve* complex. Tricuspid valve incompetence may be due to disease or abnormalities of the tricuspid *leaflets, chordae, papillary muscles,* right ventricular *myocardium, annulus,* or a *combination* of these. While many conditions can affect tricuspid valve function, acquired isolated tricuspid incompetence rarely is found without associated cardiovascular abnormalities, except following infective endocarditis or cardiac trauma.

Although the tricuspid valve functions well when the right ventricular is normal, elevations in RV diastolic volume or pulmonary artery systolic pressure commonly result in incompetence of this valve. The elevation may be transient or variable, most likely related to intermittent dilatation of the tricuspid annulus. Functional or secondary tricuspid regurgitation occurs readily in the absence of organic tricuspid valve disease, particularly in the presence of an RV pressure or volume overload. Biventricular congestive heart failure with a high right ventricular end-diastolic pressure may cause tricuspid incompetence even in the absence of severe pulmonary hypertension.

Etiology

Table 16-1 summarizes the causes of tricuspid regurgitation.

Organic or Primary Disease of the Tricuspid Valve

Rheumatic fever affects the tricuspid valve, and autopsy evidence of tricuspid valvulitis is not infrequent. Clinically apparent tricuspid disease,

Table 16-1. Etiology of Tricuspid Regurgitation

Etiology
Organic involvement of the tricuspid valve
Rheumatic valvulitis
Infective endocarditis
Trauma to the heart
Acute right ventricular infarction
Carcinoid syndrome
Tricuspid valve prolapse
Ebstein's anomaly
Functional abnormalities of the tricuspid valve
Right ventricular dilatation, acute or chronic
Pulmonary hypertension
Combination of RV volume and pressure overload

manifested as tricuspid regurgitation, tricuspid stenosis, or a combination of both lesions, is apparent in less than 20% of patients with overt rheumatic heart disease. Infective endocarditis is the most common cause of isolated tricuspid regurgitation in adults, found almost exclusively in drug abusers. Right-sided endocarditis is common in heroin addicts, occurring in 5% of this population. Cardiac trauma can produce tricuspid regurgitation. Although penetrating injuries can injure the valve, blunt chest trauma is a more common cause of tricuspid incompetence. The actual episode may have occurred months to years earlier. Steering wheel and motorcycle accidents are particularly suspect.

Right ventricular infarction resulting from acute inferior wall myocardial infarction is a recently identified cause of tricuspid regurgitation. An iatrogenic cause of tricuspid regurgitation is transvenous placement of a pacemaker in which the electrode catheter is positioned across the tricuspid valve. Carcinoid syndrome resulting from a rare serotonin-producing tumor of the intestine may result in a peculiar right heart fibrosis with the undersurface of the tricuspid and pulmonary valve leaflets adhering to the RV septal wall.

Functional or Secondary Tricuspid Regurgitation

Incompetence of the tricuspid valve resulting from RV dilation or elevation of RV systolic and diastolic pressure is the most common cause of tricuspid regurgitation in adults. Rheumatic mitral valve disease, particularly mitral stenosis, is a common cause of secondary tricuspid regurgitation.

Tricuspid regurgitation may be produced by pulmonary hypertension of other etiologies, such as primary pulmonary hypertension, major pulmonary emboli, Eisenmenger's reaction, and severe cor pulmonale. Severe left ventricular failure from cardiomyopathy or other causes frequently can be associated with an incompetent tricuspid valve, especially during periods of cardiac decompensation.

Pathophysiology

Importance of Pulmonary Artery Pressure

When considering tricuspid regurgitation, it is useful to categorize patients into those with normal pulmonary artery pressure and those with pulmonary hypertension.

Normal Pulmonary Artery Pressure

In the absence of elevation of the pulmonary artery pressure, the RV faces a pure volume overload in tricuspid regurgitation. In general, the magnitude of the valvular incompetence is less than when pulmonary hypertension is present. The normal right ventricle and the right atrium are relatively compliant; systemic venous distention is not seen in "low-pressure" tricuspid regurgitation unless the tricuspid leak is enormous or the severe RV volume overload results in RV dysfunction. Therefore, the classic tricuspid murmur and elevated jugular venous pressure with V waves may be attenuated or absent. *Practical Point: An inspiratory increase in the intensity of the systolic murmur and the amplitude of venous V wave are of great diagnostic importance in patients with low-pressure tricuspid regurgitation.* Such subjects often have no abnormal findings during expiration.

Elevated Pulmonary Artery Pressure

Tricuspid regurgitation resulting from or complicated by pulmonary hypertension tends to be more severe. Decreased compliance of the hypertrophied right ventricle augments the magnitude of the tricuspid regurgitation. In patients with rheumatic mitral valve disease or chronic congestive heart failure, tricuspid regurgitation usually is seen in subjects with mean right atrial pressures greater than 8–10 mmHg. The right ventricle in chronic severe pulmonary hypertension has an increased diastolic pressure and volume (chamber dilatation); ultimately, the tricuspid valve ring or annulus dilates.

Effects on Right Atrial Dynamics

The right atrial X descent is attenuated in mild tricuspid regurgitation and completely obliterated with moderate to severe tricuspid reflux. A systolic regurgitant V wave replaces the normal decrease in right atrial and jugular venous pressure during systole (Figures 16-1 and 16-2).

Severe tricuspid regurgitation causes the RV to dilate further; therefore, tricuspid regurgitation begets more tricuspid regurgitation. Severe tricuspid regurgitation causes retrograde systolic flow with reversal of flow in the great veins. The right atrial and jugular venous descent become sharp and steep, reflecting the rapid and voluminous diastolic right ventricular filling that takes place in the presence of an elevated right atrial pressure (see Figures 16-1 and 16-2).

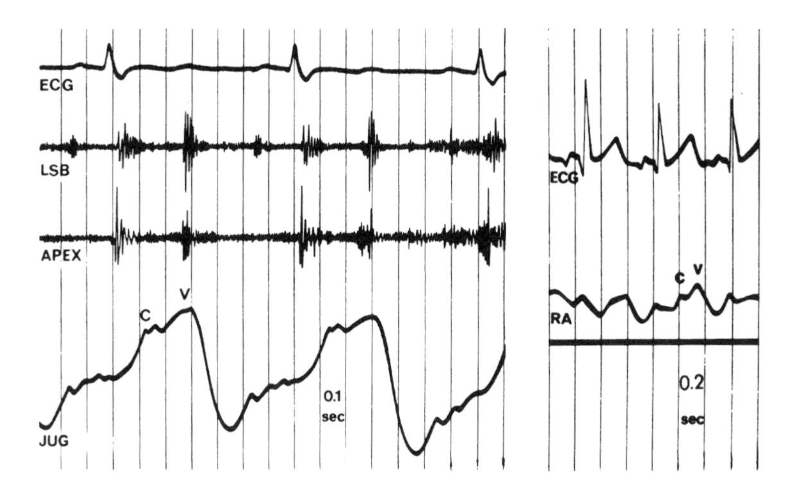

Figure 16-1. Jugular venous contour in tricuspid regurgitation. (Left) A jugular venous tracing (Jug) is shown demonstrating an enormous C-V wave with loss of the X descent. (Right) A direct right atrial (RA) tracing is shown but with a different pressure scale. Note the similarity in the waveform contour between the right atrium and the jugular venous pulse. (Reprinted with permission from Tavel ME. Phonocardiography: Clinical use with and without combined echocardiography. *Prog Cardiovasc Dis.* 1983;26:145.)

Systemic Effects

Chronic systemic venous pressure elevation may cause congestion of the liver and bowel (Table 16-2). Hepatomegaly with parenchymal dysfunction of the liver and ascites are not unusual in chronic severe tricuspid regurgitation. Decreased renal perfusion and low cardiac output lead to further fluid retention and edema.

Effects of Respiration

The normal physiologic inspiratory increase of venous return to the right heart is important in cardiac physical diagnosis when evaluating abnormalities of the tricuspid valve. If the tricuspid valve is incompetent, the larger inspiratory RV stroke volume refluxes into the right atrium. The volume and velocity of RV blood refluxing across the tricuspid valve into the right atrium therefore increases during inspi-

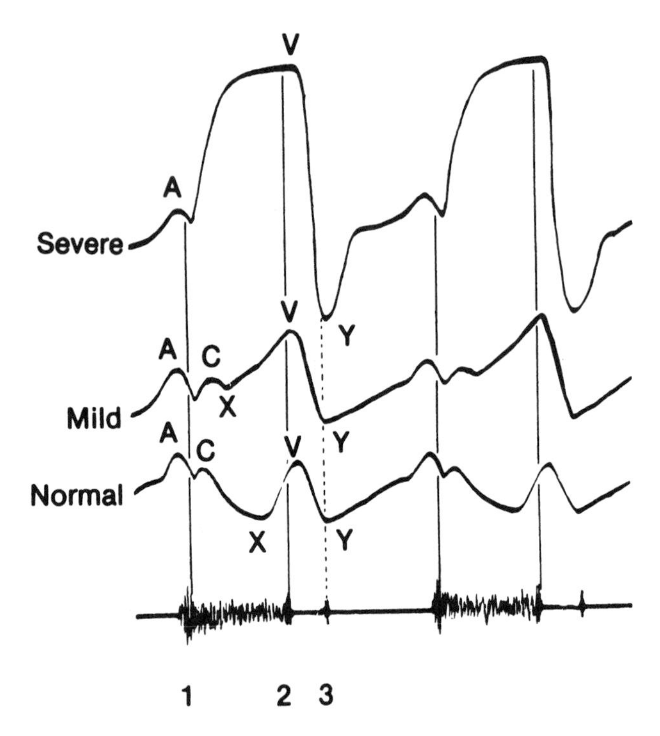

Figure 16-2. Jugular venous pulse in tricuspid regurgitation. Alterations of the venous contour in mild tricuspid regurgitation are depicted in the middle tracing. The V wave is augmented and the Y descent is more prominent; the X descent is attenuated markedly. With severe tricuspid regurgitation (top tracing), there is a plateaulike systolic regurgitant C-V wave, which in part represents "ventricularization" of the right atrial and jugular venous pulses. Note the right ventricular S_3 coinciding with the nadir of the Y descent. A normal venous pulse is depicted in the bottom.

ration. Inspiratory augmentation of regurgitant flow results in a greater amplitude (and often duration) of the jugular venous V wave as well as prominence of the murmur of tricuspid regurgitation. *Practical Point: Inspiratory augmentation of the systolic murmur is a classic physical finding in tricuspid regurgitation* (Figure 16-3).

Table 16-2. Noncardiac Manifestations of Severe Tricuspid Regurgitation

Head bob
Proptosis
Anterior motion of eyes
Engorged neck
Hepatomegaly
Pulsatile liver
Splenomegaly
Ascites
Peripheral edema
Mild icterus
Acrocyanosis
Cachexia: weight loss, muscle wasting

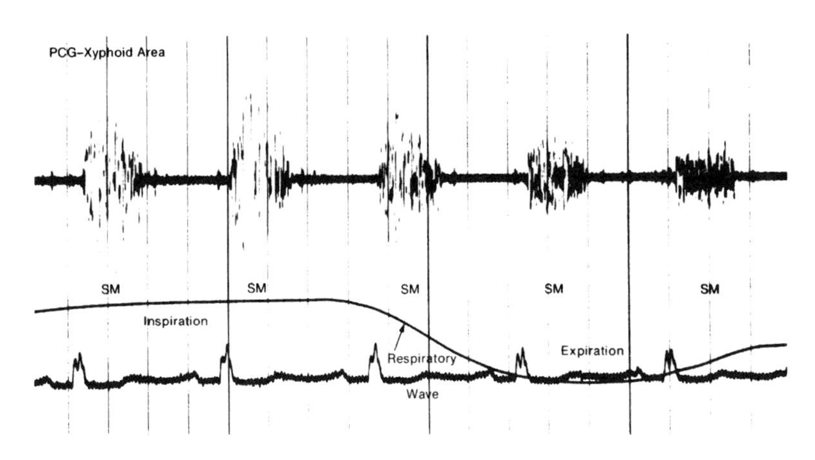

Figure 16-3. Inspiratory augmentation of the murmur of tricuspid regurgitation. Note the dramatic increase in amplitude of the systolic murmur (SM) during inspiration. Augmented right ventricular filling and a greater tricuspid regurgitant volume during inspiration produces a louder murmur. (Reprinted with permission from Delman AJ, Stein E. *Dynamic Cardiac Auscultation and Phonocardiography*. Philadelphia: WB Saunders Co.; 1979.)

Failure of Murmur to Increase in Inspiration

If the right ventricle is unable to increase its end-diastolic volume further during inspiration, there can be no additional inspiratory augmentation of regurgitant flow or murmur enhancement. This situation occurs when the degree of tricuspid regurgitation is massive and RV diastolic volume maximal or the right ventricle has failed and no longer can alter its stroke volume during the respiratory cycle. In such cases, there will be no respiratory alteration in murmur intensity.

Diastolic events such as an RV S_3 and RV S_4, a tricuspid opening snap, and a tricuspid middiastolic flow rumble also are of greater intensity during inspiration in patients with tricuspid valve disease.

Atrial Fibrillation

In chronic tricuspid regurgitation, particularly when moderately severe, atrial fibrillation is common. In some series, this is present in more than 85% of patients, most of whom have chronic valvular heart disease.

Physical Examination

General Appearance

In mild tricuspid regurgitation, there are no alterations in the physical appearance. Chronic severe tricuspid regurgitation, usually in association with pulmonary hypertension, frequently results in sustained elevation of systemic venous pressure, which can result in hepatic and renal dysfunction. Noncardiac physical findings associated with tricuspid regurgitation are listed in Table 16-2. All are related to marked elevation of the systemic venous pressure or large transmitted V waves.

The Liver

Typically, the liver is enlarged in chronic tricuspid regurgitation. The liver may be tender or hard and insensitive to palpation (cardiac cirrhosis). The liver usually is *pulsatile,* a finding frequently missed at the bedside. The low-amplitude hepatic pulsations directly reflect reversed systolic blood flow in the great veins. A pulsatile liver must be distinguished from the pulsations of a normal, dilated, or tortuous abdominal aorta. The latter are more medial, and the pulsations are directed anteriorly. Bimanual palpation of the liver can be useful in this differentiation; hepatic pulsations tend to be expansile in all directions. The more rightward and lateral in the abdomen the liver can be felt, the easier it is to distinguish a hepatic impulse from that of the abdominal aorta.

Practical Point: The low-amplitude hepatic pulsations of tricuspid regurgitation often are better seen than felt. The patient should be asked to hold his or her breath (fixing the diaphragm) in deep inspiration while the clinician carefully observes the examining fingers and hand for motion with each cardiac cycle. Close attention should be given to the hepatic motion during held inspiration. In patients with atrial fibrillation, it is more difficult to detect inspiratory augmentation because of the variability in regurgitant volume from beat to beat; nevertheless, liver pulsations should be readily detectable.

Chronic passive hepatic distention may produce low-grade jaundice and scleral icterus. Liver function tests will be deranged. A protein-losing enteropathy has been described in chronic severe tricuspid regurgitation as a result of lymphangiectasia and direct seepage of protein into the gut. The resultant depression of serum proteins further potentiates formation of edema. Splenomegaly has been observed in these patients, a direct consequence of chronic passive congestion of the systemic venous bed. The low cardiac output typical of patients with chronic tricuspid regurgitation may cause mild cyanosis of the lips, fingers, and toes. The combination of cyanosis and icterus can give some patients a sickly, sallow hue.

Fluid Retention

Most but not all subjects with chronic tricuspid regurgitation have chronic edema, which may be marked. Ascites also is common, reflecting hepatic venous and lymphatic congestion as well as renal salt and water retention.

In end-stage rheumatic heart disease or severe long-standing pulmonary hypertension, patients with tricuspid regurgitation demonstrate the muscle wasting and weight loss (cardiac cachexia) often associated with edema and ascites. Patients with severe tricuspid regurgitation and associated cardiac lesions typically have little evidence of pulmonary congestion. Such subjects can lie relatively flat without orthopnea or paroxysmal nocturnal dyspnea.

Arterial Pulse

There are no characteristic alterations of the carotid pulse in tricuspid regurgitation. The arterial pulse amplitude may be diminutive if left ventricular stroke volume is reduced.

It is easy to confuse the dramatic swelling of the jugular veins found in patients with severe tricuspid regurgitation (see later) with the arterial pulse. These pulsations (V or regurgitant waves) are systolic in timing and may be visible as well as palpable (see Figures 16-1 and 16-2). Chronic elevation of venous pressure may result in thickened jugular veins with decreased compliance; the forcefulness of the venous V wave may be surprisingly great. Such pulsations may simulate the arterial pulse of aortic regurgitation. As a general rule, large systolic jugular *venous* pulsations are more lateral in the neck and generally have a more gradual or rounded contour. The venous pulse can be obliterated by firm pressure at the base of the neck. A problem of differentiation of venous from arterial pulsations occurs only in patients with severe tricuspid regurgitation and a high mean venous pressure (see page 30 and Table 3-1).

Jugular Venous Pulse

Neck vein pulsations in tricuspid regurgitation are of extreme diagnostic importance. The diagnosis of an incompetent tricuspid valve often can be suggested prior to auscultation after a careful examination of the jugular pulse.

As the severity of tricuspid regurgitation increases in magnitude, the X descent becomes attenuated and ultimately disappears (see Figure 16-2). With increasing degrees of tricuspid reflux, a positive venous pulse wave appears during systole. This has been called an *S wave, C-V wave, V wave,* or *regurgitant wave*. It often is prominent. The regurgitant wave is systolic and approximately simultaneous with the palpable carotid arterial pulse, although its precise timing, peak, and contour are somewhat different from the arterial pulsation. The venous C-V wave has a more rounded contour and is somewhat sustained or plateaulike, in contrast to the brisk up-and-down motion of the arterial pulse (see Figures 16-1 and 16-2).

With increasing degrees of tricuspid regurgitation, the venous pulsation begins earlier in systole. The large systolic V or regurgitant wave is terminated by a sharp steep trough, the Y descent, which represents decompression of the right atrium as the tricuspid valve opens fully in early diastole (see Figure 16-2). The prominent Y descent is seen easily and actually may be more prominent than the swelling of the venous pulse (V wave) preceding the Y collapse (see Figures 16-1 and 16-2).

In most adult patients with acquired tricuspid regurgitation due to pulmonary hypertension, the mean venous pressure is elevated. Therefore, the peak of the venous systolic wave may be high; it often is necessary to examine such subjects in a semirecumbent or sitting position. With very high venous pressures, the meniscus of the venous blood column may be invisible, as the venous system is tense and distended with blood.

Effects of Respiration

The magnitude of tricuspid reflux increases as RV inflow increases during inspiration; as the right atrium distends, more blood regurgitates into the superior vena cava. This is manifest as a larger V wave, which has a higher peak and mean pressure and a more prominent Y descent during inspiration. In patients with mild to moderate tricuspid regurgitation or a large compliant right atrium, the inspiratory increase in the V wave may be a more reliable clue to the presence of tricuspid regurgitation than ausculatory changes in the systolic murmur. If severe right ventricular failure or massive tricuspid regurgitation is present, the right ventricle may be unable to fill any further and an inspiratory increase in venous pressure will not be noted.

Atrial Fibrillation

The arrhythmia of atrial fibrillation may cause difficulty in diagnosing tricuspid regurgitation, as the varying cycle lengths alter the degree of tricuspid reflex on a beat-to-beat basis. Respiratory alterations in the level of the venous pressure and V wave height may be impossible to detect.

Ancillary Signs

On occasion, severe chronic tricuspid regurgitation produces some remarkable findings related to the huge venous V waves and high systemic venous pressure. Pulsations of the head (right-to-left head bob with each cardiac cycle), eyeballs, and earlobes have been observed in major tricuspid regurgitation. The eyes also may be slightly proptotic from chronically elevated venous pressure. *Practical Point: Subtle systolic motion of the earlobes or lateral swelling of the neck with each heart beat are common clues to the presence of severe tricuspid regurgitation* (Figure 16-4).

For optimal assessment of the venous pressure and contour, one must inspect the neck carefully, using tangential lighting and various degrees of elevation of the head (see Figure 3-2). Chronic distention of the systemic veins may render the venous valves incompetent, allowing transmission of the systolic V wave to the periphery of the venous tree. This may result in pulsations of the veins on the backs of

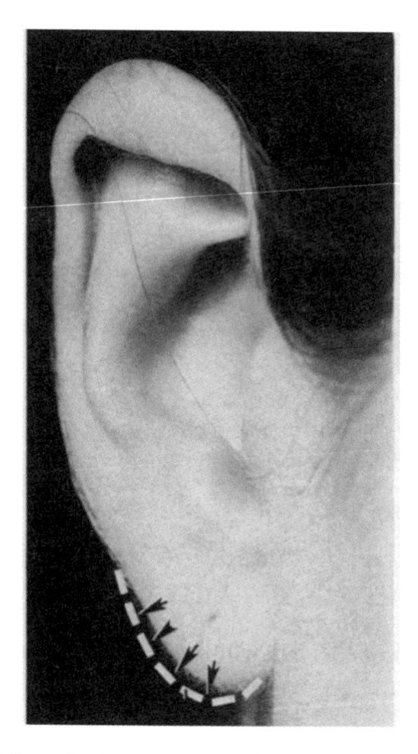

Figure 16-4. Earlobe pulsations in tricuspid regurgitation. In severe tricuspid regurgitation, the jugular venous pressure is elevated markedly and the large V waves may be difficult to discern. Careful inspection of the earlobe with the patient in a 30–90° position may reveal subtle lateral pulsations of the large systolic V waves in the right atrium throughout the proximal venous system.

the hands, arms, or legs, which are seen when the extremity is elevated to the level of actual mean venous pressure.

A "Normal" Venous Pulse

On occasion, the jugular venous pressure and pulse wave contour may be normal in tricuspid regurgitation, particularly in patients in sinus rhythm who have a mild degree of tricuspid reflux. On rare occasions, even severe tricuspid regurgitation can be associated with a minimal abnormality of right atrial pressure.

One can augment or bring out an abnormal V wave in equivocal cases. Anything that increases return to the right heart augments the magnitude of tricuspid regurgitation, such as leg elevation, slow deep inspiration, or mild exercise (e.g., sit-ups). The hepatojugular reflux maneuver (see Figure 3-3 and pages 29–30) also may be helpful in the detection of tricuspid regurgitation; sustained abdominal pressure results in selective augmentation of the venous V wave and the systolic murmur in tricuspid regurgitation.

Precordial Motion

In the absence of pulmonary hypertension, tricuspid regurgitation causes prominent systolic unloading of the RV. Parasternal activity reveals a retraction wave during late systole. Following a brisk early systolic outward motion, during the remainder of systole, the RV pulls away from the chest wall. An exaggerated early diastolic RV filling wave may be palpable (RV S_3). In subjects with pulmonary hypertension, a systolic upward RV impulse typically is present; this is a low-amplitude, sustained parasternal lift or heave (see Chapter 4).

Palpable right ventricular activity in tricuspid regurgitation thus reflects the level of pulmonary artery pressure, the RV size, and the severity of tricuspid regurgitation. An outward systolic impulse is felt in most instances; it is brief and early systolic in the nonpressure overloaded right ventricle and likely to be sustained when there is major pulmonary hypertension. When the RV is large, as often the case with chronic tricuspid regurgitation, the precordial activity may produce a rocking or seesaw motion. The left anterior chest and LV apex retract as the medial RV area, adjacent to lower left sternal border, moves anteriorly and then retracts during mid- to late systole. A greatly enlarged RV may occupy the usual apex area, actually pushing the LV posterolaterally in the thorax, where it no longer is palpable on the chest wall.

Heart Sounds

First Heart Sound

There are no important alterations of S_1 in tricuspid regurgitation.

Second Heart Sound

As severe pulmonary hypertension is a common cause of tricuspid regurgitation, an accentuated P_2 often is present and may be widely transmitted over the precordium. If severe RV failure is present, RV ejection will be prolonged and the stroke volume relatively fixed during respiration; S_2 will be widely split both in inspiration and expiration. This can simulate the fixed splitting of an atrial septal defect.

Third Heart Sound

An audible RV S_3 often can be heard in tricuspid regurgitation (Figure 16-5). The S_3 may reflect the excessive volume of blood crossing the tricuspid valve in early diastole or RV decompensation associated with a large RV end-diastolic volume and decreased ejection fraction. Right-sided ventricular filling sounds (S_3 and S_4) typically are louder during inspiration and wane with expiration. Such sounds may be audible only in inspiration.

A right ventricular S_3 is heard best at the lower left sternal border and inaudible at the LV apex. However, if the RV is large and occupies the apical region in the left thorax, an RV S_3 may be readily mistaken for an S_3 of left ventricular origin.

The RV S_3 often is associated with high RV diastolic pressures and may be high pitched, simulating a pericardial knock or a tricuspid opening snap. The pericardial knock of constrictive pericarditis is an unusually prominent, early, and high-pitched RV filling sound (i.e., an S_3). As with mitral regurgitation, severe tricuspid regurgitation with a large regurgitant fraction may produce a brief diastolic flow rumble (see Figure 16-5B). This murmur increases with inspiration.

Fourth Heart Sound

A right-sided atrial gallop may be heard in patients with acute-onset tricuspid regurgitation. This is similar to the left-sided S_4 found in patients with acute mitral regurgitation (see Chapter 13). In such cases, the right ventricle and the right atrium usually are of normal size; the regurgitant volume load results in vigorous right atrial contraction and produces a large increase in end-diastolic flow and

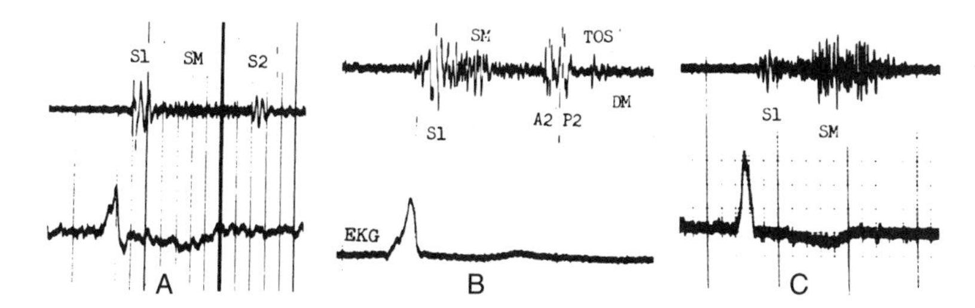

Figure 16-5. Murmurs of tricuspid regurgitation. These phonocardiograms were taken at the lower left sternal border in three individuals with tricuspid insufficiency. (A) The soft holosystolic murmur has a plateaulike configuration. (B) The murmur peaks in early systole, although sound vibrations appear to extend to A_2. Note the tricuspid opening snap, followed by a diastolic flow murmur. (C) This tricuspid murmur has late systolic accentuation. SM = systolic murmur; TOS = tricuspid opening snap; DM = diastolic murmur. (Reprinted with permission from Hultgren HN, Hancock EW, Cohn KE. Auscultation in mitral and tricuspid valvular disease. *Prog Cardiovas Dis.* 1968;10:298.)

pressure in the right ventricle. Acute tricuspid regurgitation is likely to occur in a drug addict with tricuspid valve endocarditis or a patient with traumatic rupture of a tricuspid valve cusp.

The right ventricular S_4 may be loud. It is heard best at the lower left sternal border at the fourth to fifth interspace and augments with inspiration.

Systolic Click

Early

Patients with severe pulmonary hypertension may have a pulmonary artery ejection sound, often decreasing with inspiration and heard best at the upper left sternal border (see Figure 7-4). The respiratory variation of the click (decreases with inspiration) should differentiate this sound transient from an aortic ejection click or prominently split S_1.

Mid to Late

Tricuspid valve prolapse usually is not diagnosed on auscultation, although it may be detected on echocardiography. Nevertheless, the prominence of a mid- to late-systolic click at the lower left sternal border that becomes louder and later during inspiration should raise the suspicion of tricuspid valve prolapse.

Murmurs

The classic murmur of tricuspid regurgitation is holosystolic, increases with inspiration, and is best heard at the fourth and fifth interspace at the lower left sternal border. The tricuspid regurgitation murmur usually is not very loud and may be extremely variable in character. Frequently, it is missed by physicians who do not see many patients with cardiac disease, and it often is not recognized by experienced cardiologists. *Practical Point: The correct diagnosis often will be made only if the examiner specifically looks for the subtle clues of tricuspid regurgitation.* The possibility of tricuspid regurgitation should be considered actively in any patient who shows evidence of pulmonary hypertension.

Contour

The usual tricuspid regurgitation murmur has an even, pansystolic configuration extending to S_2 (see Figures 16-2, 16-3, and 16-5A). The murmur's shape may change during the respiratory cycle (see Figure 16-3). However, it is common for the murmur to wane in late systole (see Figures 16-3, 16-5B, and 16-5C), often with early to midsystolic accentuation (see Figures 16-3 and 16-5B).

On occasion, a tricuspid regurgitation murmur that tapers off in late systole is not pansystolic; this type of murmur is most likely to occur in mild tricuspid regurgitation, in the absence of pulmonary hypertension, or in acute-onset tricuspid regurgitation. When the tricuspid valve is incompetent and the RV has a normal systolic pressure, the volume and velocity of blood refluxing into the right atrium in late systole is small. In such cases, the tricuspid murmur commonly is soft and short, and the correct diagnosis easily is missed. One may have to rely on *respiratory variation* in the murmur intensity and the *ancillary signs* of tricuspid regurgitation (jugular venous pulse, pulsatile liver) to make the appropriate diagnosis.

Intensity

The murmur of tricuspid regurgitation seldom is very loud and usually of grade 2 or 2–3 intensity. Tricuspid regurgitation has been documented to be acoustically silent in many patients, particularly those with a mild to moderate degree of reflux. Minimal regurgitation is a "normal" echocardiographic finding. Silent tricuspid regurgitation is more likely to occur with normal RV systolic pressure, such as that found with traumatic or infectious damage to a previously normal valve. Making the proper diagnosis in such cases is not easy. In some patients, the murmur is heard only during inspiration, which can be misleading, as it may simulate a pulmonary or pericardial process. Variation in inspiratory intensity may be difficult to detect when the tricuspid murmur is very loud. It is not uncommon for the murmur of tricuspid regurgitation to augment 1–2 grades in intensity during inspiration (see Figure 16-3).

Frequency

The typical tricuspid regurgitation murmur is of medium frequency but on occasion can be rough and raspy. High-frequency murmurs of tricuspid regurgitation are not common. The murmur may appear to be higher pitched at sites away from the area of maximal intensity. It is best to use both the bell and diaphragm of the stethoscope when listening for tricuspid regurgitation.

Tricuspid Honk or Whoop

Tricuspid regurgitation rarely can be associated with a vibratory, high-pitched whoop, which usually demonstrates a prominent inspiratory increase. This tricuspid honk usually is intermittent and has been associated with severe pulmonary hypertension. Tricuspid valve prolapse is likely to be an etiologic factor.

Location and Radiation

The tricuspid regurgitation murmur is heard best over the right ventricular area at the lower left sternal edge at the fourth to fifth interspace. The murmur may radiate into both the right and left chest for a short distance. Transmission to the lower right sternal area is common, and one should listen carefully at the lower right sternal border whenever tricuspid regurgitation is suspected. When loud, the murmur also may be heard at the upper left sternal edge. Soft tricuspid murmurs may be well localized to a small area of the lower left sternal border.

When the RV is very large, the murmur may be heard at both the left lower sternal edge and the cardiac apex, which may be formed by the dilated right ventricular chamber. In such cases, the murmur may be equally loud at the mid-left chest and sternal edge, but it will never be loudest at the apex. It is easy to mistake the apical murmur of tricuspid regurgitation for mitral regurgitation. If the apical murmur is solely tricuspid in origin, it does not radiate into the axilla. Inspiratory augmentation should be carefully assessed. Careful inching of the stethoscope from the lower left sternal border to the apex can be very helpful.

Tricuspid regurgitation murmurs often are easily detected at the xiphoid and subxiphoid areas, particularly in patients with large chests or chronic obstructive pulmonary disease. *Practical Point: Whenever tricuspid regurgitation is suspected, listen carefully for murmur radiation to the right lower sternal border, xiphoid region, and over the superior aspect of the liver.*

Respiratory Alteration

The inspiratory increase in the intensity of the murmur of tricuspid regurgitation, known as *Carvallo's sign*, is a well-known phenomenon (see Figure 16-3). Respiratory alteration, however, is frequently full grade and may be a subtle finding. For optimal detection of respiratory variation, it may be useful to auscultate several centimeters *away from* the point of peak murmur intensity. With very loud murmurs minor respiratory alterations in intensity may be difficult to detect.

One must be sure the patient is breathing deeply and smoothly with no forced respiration or inadvertent Valsalva maneuver. The subject should breathe somewhat more deeply than usual in a continuous fashion.

In patients with a soft murmur, inspiration may increase the grade dramatically for only one or two beats. Rarely, the systolic murmur will be heard only during inspiration while diastole remains silent. *Practical Point: For optimal auscultation, listen for respiratory variation over many respiratory cycles and focus on phasic alterations in peak intensity of the systolic murmur.*

Hepatojugular Reflux

The use of the hepatojugular reflux maneuver recently has been shown to be helpful in identifying tricuspid murmurs. Firm upward pressure with the hand over the right upper quadrant of the abdomen for 10–15 sec accentuates the murmur of tricuspid regurgitation (see pages 29–30 and Figure 3-3). The maneuver is especially useful in patients with only mild to moderate tricuspid regurgitation and in the absence of pulmonary hypertension where Carvallo's sign is equivocal or not present. The tricuspid murmur typically increases in loudness for four to six beats.

Atrial Fibrillation

The changing cycle lengths in atrial fibrillation cause the intensity of the tricuspid murmur to vary from beat to beat, being loudest after long cycles. Respiratory variation is extremely difficult or even impossible to detect in patients with this arrhythmia. *Practical Point: Do not conclude tricuspid regurgitation is absent because respiratory variation in the systolic murmur cannot be demonstrated in such patients.* In general, it is not productive to focus on detection of inspiratory augmentation in patients with atrial fibrillation suspected of having tricuspid regurgitation.

Failure to Change with Respiration

In some instances, there is no detectable or consistent respiratory alteration in intensity of the tricuspid regurgitation murmur (Table 16-3). The hepatojugular reflux maneuver should be tried in such cases. This situation is more likely with mild tricuspid regurgitation and normal RV systolic pressure or, conversely, with tricuspid regurgitation associated with severe RV dysfunction and right heart failure. *Practical Point: Always have the patient sit or stand during auscultation when tricuspid regurgitation is suspected but respiratory variation is absent.* The decrease in right heart volume and diastolic pressure caused by the diminished return in the upright posture may allow the RV to vary its stroke volume somewhat during respiration with a resultant increase in murmur intensity during inspiration.

Changes with Various Maneuvers

The murmur of tricuspid regurgitation can be affected by factors other than respiration (Table 16-4). Anything that increases right heart return, such as elevation of the legs, squatting, the hepatojugular reflux maneuver, Müller's maneuver (inhalation with the glottis closed), or exercise will augment the systolic murmur.

Table 16-3. Conditions Associated with Failure of the Tricuspid Regurgitation Murmur to Augment with Inspiration

Mild or trivial tricuspid regurgitation, usually normal right ventricular pressure
Severe right ventricular dilatation or failure
Atrial fibrillation
Very loud murmur

Table 16-4. Factors Affecting the Loudness of the Murmur of Tricuspid Regurgitation

Increased murmur intensity caused by increased right heart filling
Inspiration
Hepatojugular reflux maneuver
Leg elevation
Squatting
Müller's maneuver
Mild exercise
Volume overload or decompensated RV failure
Valsalva maneuver, release phase (immediate)
Decreased murmur intensity caused by decreased right heart filling
Expiration
Standing
Sitting
Valsalva maneuver, strain phase
Nitroglycerin
Diuresis or hypovolemia

Variability

The clinical picture of tricuspid regurgitation may vary from day to day, particularly in the "secondary" or functional variants. The variation in the signs of tricuspid regurgitation is due to alterations in cardiovascular hemodynamics; the level of pulmonary artery pressure and the degree of RV dilatation and dysfunction act as important variables that can change from day to day. In patients with pulmonary hypertension and RV failure, intracardiac and pulmonary pressure may fluctuate considerably, depending on the status of intra- and extravascular volume, the level of physical activity, and cardiac rate and rhythm. Tricuspid regurgitation commonly is present when such patients present in a decompensated state. Severe RV failure may cause the tricuspid regurgitation to be completely missed on initial examination due to marked distention of the venous system (failure to observe V wave) and absence of respiratory change in the murmur (presence of atrial fibrillation or severe right ventricular failure). After therapy, the tricuspid regurgitation may become clinically evident. When treatment is maximal (e.g., conversion to normal sinus rhythm, following substantial diuresis, or rate control in atrial fibrillation), the tricuspid regurgitation may resolve completely.

Diastolic Murmur

An early middiastolic tricuspid murmur may be noted in patients with substantial tricuspid regurgitation (see Figure 16-5B). This murmur represents diastolic flow across the open tricuspid valve. The murmur usually is of medium to low frequency. It is heard best at the lower left sternal border (fourth to fifth interspace) and follows the tricuspid opening snap or S_3, if present. It commonly augments with inspiration.

Differential Diagnosis

The murmur of tricuspid regurgitation often is missed, particularly when there are other obvious causes of a heart murmur. The murmur may be thought to be innocent or confused with mitral regurgitation. Associated cardiac lesions may confuse the issue; many clinicians fail to think of tricuspid regurgitation as a diagnostic possibility. The frequent, atypical presentation of the tricuspid regurgitation murmur (not holosystolic, no increase with inspiration) also is a problem. Tricuspid regurgitation will be diagnosed appropriately far more often if the physician has an expectant attitude, particularly in any patient suspected of having pulmonary hypertension.

Mitral Regurgitation

The holosystolic murmur of mitral regurgitation occasionally may radiate toward the sternum. If the heart is not large, the murmur may be prominent in the tricuspid area. Respiratory variation and augmented venous V waves indicate tricuspid regurgitation; in the absence of overt congestive heart failure, the inability of the holosystolic murmur to increase with inspiration favors mitral regurgitation. In atrial fibrillation, the respiratory variation of the murmur readily may be missed. Patients with RV dilatation present a different problem because tricuspid regurgitation readily may be mistaken for mitral regurgitation when the right ventricle forms the cardiac apex. The absence of murmur radiation into the axillary region and the presence of respiratory variation are crucial diagnostic points favoring tricuspid origin of the murmur.

It is not uncommon for a patient to have both mitral and tricuspid regurgitation. In such instances, one of the valve lesions may be missed on auscultation. Typically, the holosystolic murmur will wane and then increase in intensity as the stethoscope is inched from the lower left sternal border toward the cardiac apex or vice versa. Respiratory variation will be audible medially but not laterally in the left chest. When the tricuspid regurgitation murmur is loud, it may be extremely difficult to be sure whether coexisting mitral regurgitation is present.

Ventricular Septal Defect

Both a ventricular septal defect and tricuspid regurgitation produce a holosystolic murmur at the lower left sternal edge but rarely is differentiating these two conditions a problem. Ventricular septal defects usually are found in children and only infrequently in young adults. There is no inspiratory augmentation of the murmur, and the jugular venous pulse is normal in patients with VSD. Furthermore, the VSD murmur is likely to be quite loud. In acute myocardial infarction complicated by a ventricular septal defect, the differential between the two lesions may be difficult or even impossible if there is no respiratory change in the murmur.

Functional Murmurs

When the tricuspid regurgitation murmur is short (normal pulmonary artery systolic pressure, acute tricuspid regurgitation) and does not extend to S_2, it readily may simulate an ejection murmur of nonspecific nature. The location is lower (fourth to fifth interspace at the left sternal edge) than the usual flow murmur. Respiratory variation is the most important discriminator. Functional murmurs tend to soften in inspiration, if at all.

References

Abrams J. Approach to the patient with heart murmurs. In: Kelley W, ed. *Textbook of Internal Medicine*. 3rd ed. Philadelphia: Lippincott-Raven; 1997;337–342.

Abrams J. *Synopsis of Cardiac Physical Diagnosis*. Philadelphia: Lea & Febiger; 1989.

Abrams J. *Essentials of Cardiac Physical Diagnosis*. Philadelphia: Lea & Febiger; 1987.

Altman CA, Nihil MR, Bricker JT. *Pediatric Cardiac Auscultation*. CD-ROM. Hagerstown, MD: Lippincott, Williams & Wilkins; 2000.

Chizner MA. Bedside diagnosis of the acute myocardial infarction and its complications. *Curr Probl Cardiol*. 1982;7:1.

Constant J. *Bedside Cardiology*. 4th ed. Boston: Little, Brown; 1993.

Craige E, Millward DK. Diastolic and continuous murmurs. *Prog Cardiovasc Dis*. 1971;14:38.

Crawford MH, O'Rourke RA. A systematic approach to bedside differentiation of cardiac murmurs and abnormal sounds. *Curr Probl Cardiol*. 1977;1:1.

Criley JM. *Beyond Heart Sounds: The Interactive Cardiac Exam*. Vol. 1. CD-ROM. Hagerstown, MD: Lippincott, Williams & Wilkins; 1999-2001.

Criley JM, Criley D, Zalace C. *The Physiological Origins of Heart Sounds and Murmurs: The Unique Interactive Guide to Cardiac Diagnosis*. CD-ROM. Hagerstown MD: Lippincott, Williams & Wilkins; 1996.

Delman AJ, Stein E. *Dynamic Cardiac Auscultation and Phonocardiography*. Philadelphia: WB Saunders Co.; 1979.

Grewe K, Crawford MH, O'Rourke RA. Differentiation of cardiac murmurs by dynamic auscultation. *Curr Probl Cardiol*. 1988;13.

Harvey WP. Innocent vs. significant murmurs. *Curr Prob Cardiol*. 1976;1:1.

Horwitz LD, Groves LD, eds. *Signs and Symptoms in Cardiology*. Philadelphia: Lippincott; 1985.

Hultgren HN, Hancock EW, Cohn KE. Auscultation. Part I: mitral and tricuspid valve disease. *Prog Cardio Dis.* 1968;10:298.

Leatham A. *Auscultation of the Heart and Phonocardiography.* 2nd ed. Edinburgh: Churchill Livingstone; 1975.

Lembo NJ, Dell'Italia LJ, Crawford MH, O'Rourke RA. Bedside diagnosis of systolic murmurs. *N Engl J Med.* 1988;318:1572.

Lembo NJ, Dell'Italia LJ, Crawford MH, O'Rourke RA. Diagnosis of left-sided regurgitant murmurs by transient arterial occlusion: a new maneuver using blood pressure cuffs. *Ann Intern Med.* 1986;105:368.

Leon DF, Shaver JA, eds. Physiologic Principles of Heart Sounds and Murmurs. American Heart Association Monograph No. 46, 1975.

Perloff JK. *Clinical Recognition of Congenital Heart Disease.* 4th ed. Philadelphia: WB Saunders Co.; 1994.

Perloff JK. *Physical Examination of the Heart and Circulation.* Philadelphia: WB Saunders Co.; 1982.

Ravin A. *Auscultation of the Heart.* 3rd ed. Chicago: Year Book; 1976.

Reddy PS, Shaver JA, Leonard JJ. Cardiac systolic murmurs: pathophysiology and differential diagnosis. *Prog Cardiovasc Dis.* 1971;14:1.

Roberts WC. *Adult Congenital Heart Disease.* Philadelphia: FA Davis; 1986.

Shaver JA, Salerni R, Reddy PS. Normal and abnormal heart sounds in cardiac diagnosis. Part I: systolic sounds. *Curr Probl Cardiol.* 1985;10:1.

Shaver JA, Salerni R, Reddy PS. Normal and abnormal heart sounds in cardiac diagnosis. Part II: diastolic sounds. *Curr Probl Cardiol.* 1985;10:1.

Smith ND, Raizada V, Abrams J. Auscultation of the normally functioning prosthetic valve. *Ann Intern Med.* 1981;96:594.

Tavel ME. *Clinical Phonocardiography and External Pulse Recording.* 4th ed. Chicago: Year Book; 1985.

Tavel ME. Phonocardiography: clinical use with and without combined echocardiography. *Prog Cardiovasc Dis.* 1983;26:145.

Wooley CF. Rediscovery of the tricuspid valve. *Curr Probl Cardiol.* 1981;6:1.

Wooley CF. Intracardiac phonocardiography. *Circulation.* 1978;57:1039.

Index

M